Olfa ZOUKAR
Dr Wiem Ben Slamia

Twisting appendices :

Olfa ZOUKAR
Dr Wiem Ben Slamia

Twisting appendices :

The experience of the Monastir maternity and neonatology center

ScienciaScripts

Imprint

Cover image: www.ingimage.com

This book is a translation from the original published under ISBN 978-3-8381-4918-9.

Publisher:
Sciencia Scripts
is a trademark of
Dodo Books Indian Ocean Ltd. and OmniScriptum S.R.L publishing group

120 High Road, East Finchley, London, N2 9ED, United Kingdom
Str. Armeneasca 28/1, office 1, Chisinau MD-2012, Republic of Moldova, Europe
Printed at: see last page
ISBN: 978-620-7-30119-5

Contents

1 INTRODUCTION

adnexal torsion is a serious gynaecological emergency that threatens the prognosis of fertility. It is seen in 3% of patients presenting with acute pelvic pain (1). It is defined as torsion of the ovary, fallopian tube or both around the infundibulopelvic and utero-ovarian ligaments (2). This rotation compromises the ovarian pedicle, which may lead to ovarian infarction, resulting in necrosis if consultation or diagnosis is delayed (3). The presence of an ovarian mass of at least 5 cm is the main risk factor for torsion(4). Isolated torsion of the tube is possible but exceptional (5). The age range of patients is wide, from pre-menarche to post-menopause, although most cases occur in women of reproductive age (6,7).

Early diagnosis of torsion is crucial and can prevent necrosis of the adnexa and subsequent fertility problems (8). Delayed consultation, and above all delayed or difficult diagnosis, compromises the prognosis of adnexal torsion (9), as it is often difficult to make a precise preoperative diagnosis of adnexal torsion due to its polymorphous clinical symptoms and the absence of specific biological and radiological signs (10,11). The multitude of differential diagnoses with other gynaecological and surgical emergencies makes diagnosis even more difficult (12).

Ultrasound is the radiological examination of first choice (13), but it has limitations and the results reported in the literature are often inconsistent (10,14). Ultrasound findings commonly include an enlarged ovary with hyperechogenic stroma and peripheral arrangement of follicles, and usually the site of a cystic mass (15). Accurate ultrasound diagnosis of adnexal torsion has been reported in 23% to 81% of women (11), and the performance of Doppler for studying adnexal vascularisation is controversial (16). Normal arterial flow on ultrasound does not exclude ovarian torsion, and suspicion must remain in the case of a cystic mass (17). Thus, adnexal torsion is suspected preoperatively in only 23-70.8% of cases (11,18) and up to 50% of surgeries performed for suspected adnexal torsion in young women with acute pelvic pain do not reveal adnexal torsion (18).

When the diagnosis of adnexal torsion is strongly suggested, conservative laparoscopic treatment is currently the approach of choice, except in the case of a mass suspected of malignancy or torsion in a menopausal woman (19).

On the basis of these findings, we carried out this retrospective study of 100 cases in our department of any woman presenting to our emergency department with acute pelvic pain in whom adnexal torsion was suspected. We set ourselves the following objectives:

- To determine the various clinical and para-clinical signs of adnexal torsion and the prognostic factors involved.
- Establish a clinico-biological, radiological and intraoperative comparison of patients presenting with adnexal torsion.

2 MATERIALS AND METHODS

1. Type and location of study

This is a retrospective, descriptive and analytical, mono-centric study carried out in the gynecology department of the Monastir maternity and neonatology centre (CMNM), over a 5-year period from 01/01/2017 to 31/01/2022.

2. Study population

2.1. Inclusion criteria

All women who presented to our CMNM Obstetric Gynecology service with acute pelvic painë and underwent urgent surgery for suspected adnexal torsion.

2.2. Exclusion criteria

Patients with lost, incomplete or unusable records were excluded from the study.

3. Data collection

The data required for our study were collected from hospital records, operative reports, hospitalisation registers and anatomopathology registers.

For each patient, we drew up an individual analysis grid (**appendix 1**) designed for the purposes of the study.

Each sheet is structured around the following themes:

3.1. Clinical data

- **Epidemiological data (**age, marital status, hormonal status, medical and surgical history).
- **Obstetrical antecedents (**gestite, parity, abortion, gravidopuerperal status, number of cesarean sections, method of contraception).
- **Gynecological antecedents (**menstrual cycle phase, ovarian cyst, cystectomy, adnexal torsion, ovulation induction, tubal ligation, hysterectomy).
- **Clinical examination (**previous similar episode, time between onset of pain and emergency consultation, semiological signs of pain, signs associated with pain, abdominal and gynaecological examination).

3.2. Radiological data

- Ultrasound signs of adnexal torsion :
- Ovary increases in size
- Abnormal position of the tender
- Hyperechogenic stroma
- Peripheral arrangement of follicles
- Reduced or absent colour Doppler vascularisation
- Tourbillon sign search

- CT scan (if done): look for signs of adnexal torsion (same as ultrasound)

3.3. Biological data

Plasma level of the в chain of human chorionic gonadotropic hormone (beta HCG).

Blood count (CBC)

C-Reactive Protein (CRP)

3.4. The surgical procedures involved

- Type of operation: crelioscopy or laparotomy
- Operative findings: presence or absence of torsion of the adnexa (around its axis by at least 360°)
- Type of treatment: conservative or radical
- Preventing recidivism

3.5. Anatomopathological study

3.6. Post-therapeutic follow-up

3.7. Diagnostic differentials

4. Statistical analysis

All data entry and statistical analysis were carried out using Microsoft Office Excel 2019 and IBMSPSS.

4.1. Descriptive section

For qualitative variables, frequencies are presented as percentages.

For quantitative variables, the distribution of data was studied using skewness and kurtosis coefficients and tests of normality. The variables are presented as means ± standard deviation in the case of a normal distribution and as medians [25eme - 75eme] in the opposite case.

4.2. Analytical part

Fisher's exact test or Pearson's Chi-squared test were used to determine the univariate association of various parameters with surgically confirmed adnexal torsion. The Student's t test was used to compare means and the Mann Whitney test to compare means. A binary logistic regression analysis was performed to calculate the odds ratio and 95% confidence interval for the association of the different parameters with adnexal torsion. A p-value < 0.05 was considered statistically significant.

5. Bibliographical research

Bibliographic research was carried out by consulting computerised bibliographic databases (PubMed, Science Direct, Cochrane Library, Google Scholar) as well as encyclopaedias and postgraduate courses.

6. Ethical considerations and conflicts of interest

In this work, we have respected professional secrecy and patient anonymity and declare that we have no conflict of interest.

3 RESULTS

I. Epidemiological study :

1. Overall frequency :

During the study period, we counted :

- Four hundred and eight cases of ovarian tumours were operated on, 66 of which were twisted, representing a frequency of 16.17%.
- Four hundred and eighty-two gynaecological emergencies, including 106 patients, presented with adnexal torsion, which was surgically confirmed in 66 patients, a frequency of 13.69% (Figure 1).

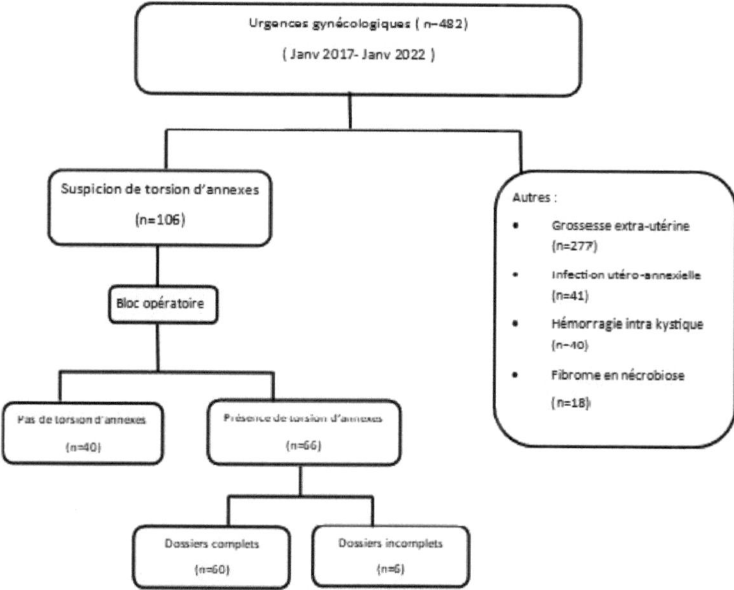

Figure 1. Flow chart of different gynaecological emergencies

2. Annual prevalence

The prevalence of torsion was around 11 cases per year (Table I).

Table I: Prevalence of adnexal torsion per year

Year	Workforce	Percentage (%)
2017	7	10,6
2018	18	27,2
2019	16	24,2
2020	11	16,7
2021	12	18,2

2022	2		3
Total	66	100	

II. Clinical data

Our clinical study included 60 women with a confirmed diagnosis of adnexal torsion with complete data.

1. Patient profile

1.1. Age

The mean age of our patients was 25.92±9.09 years, with extremes ranging from 13 to 53 years (Figure 2).

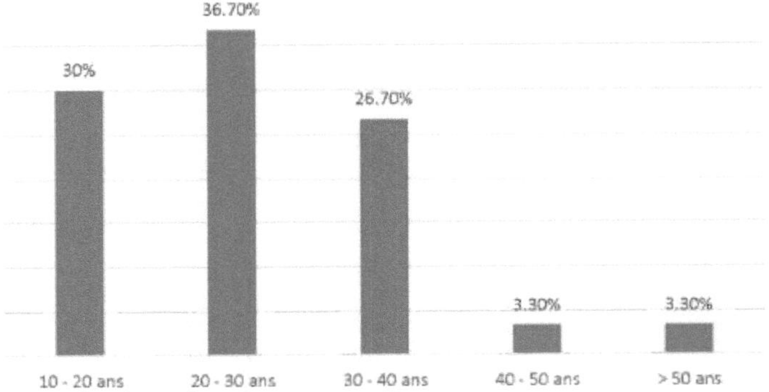

Figure 2. Distribution of patients according to age

1.2 Hormonal status

Age distribution showed a clear predominance of women of childbearing age (93%), with a peak between the ages of 20 and 30.

We noted 2 cases of menopausal women and 2 cases of pre-pubertal women (Figure 3).

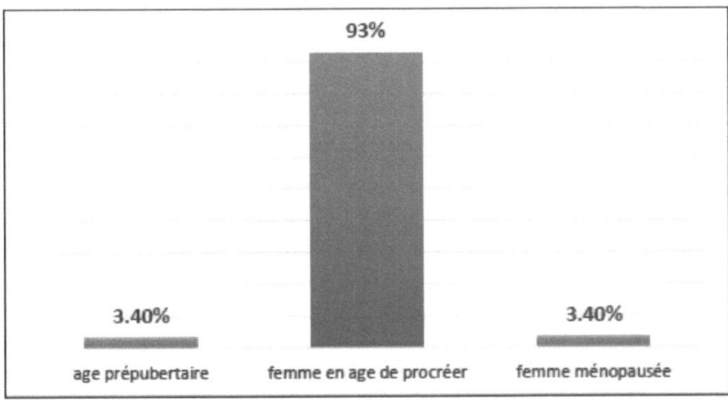

Figure 3. Hormone status of patients

1.3. Civil status

- Two-thirds of our patients, i.e. 37 cases, were single (61.7%), 4 of whom were women.

cases were of paediatric age (<= 16 years).

- The remaining third, 23 cases, were married women (38.3%) (Figure

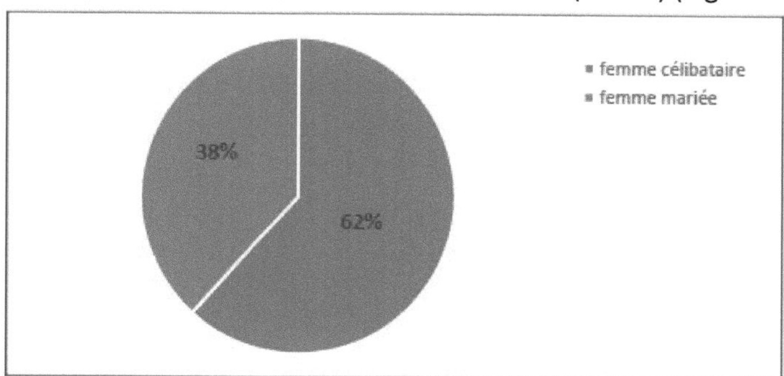

Figure 4. Marital status of patients

1.4. Pathological antecedents

The medical, surgical and gynaecological-obstetric pathological antecedents of our patients were as follows (Table II):

- The presence of a previous ovarian cyst in 8 patients (13.3% of cases).
- Previous cystectomy in 4 patients (6.7% of cases)
- A history of adnexal torsion in 1 patient.
- Previous cesarean section in 5 patients (8.3% of cases).

Table II: Patient history

Background	**Workforce**	**Percentage (%)**
Medical		
ACFA	1	1.7
Asthma	1	1.7
Hypothyroidism	1	1.7
Gastroduodenal ulcer	1	1.7
Surgical		
Appendectomy	1	1.7
Gyneco-Obstetric		
Cesarean section	5	8.3
History of ovarian cysts	8	13.3
Previous cystectomy	4	6.7
History of adnexal torsion	1	1.7

Intake of ovulation	1	1.7
Contraception by IUD	4	6.7
Tubal ligation	1	1.7
Total hysterectomy	1	1.7

1.5. Gestite-Parite

The average management was 1.32 with extremes ranging from 0 to 8. The average parity was 0.88, with extremes ranging from 0 to 6. Thirty-nine patients (65%) were nulliparous (Figure 5).

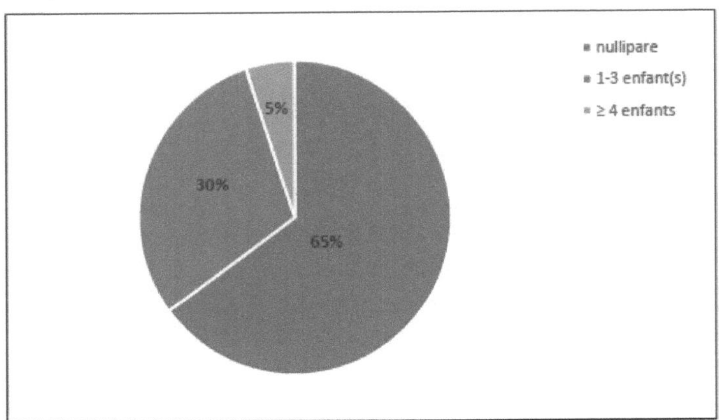

Figure 5: Parity of patients as a percentage

1.6. Pregnancy and childbirth

In our series, we noted 4 cases of pregnancy associated with adnexal torsion:

- two cases of pregnancy in the 1er trimester, one of which was induced by TSI
- two cases of spontaneous pregnancy at 24 and 26 days' gestation.

We have not noted any cases of adnexal torsion during the 3eme trimester or post partum.

1.7. Cycle phase

The date of the last menstrual period was recorded in 31 cases, with a distribution of the phases of the menstrual cycle as follows (Figure 6):

- 15 women consulted during the follicular phase (48.4%)
- 4 women consulted during the ovulatory period (12.9%)
- 12 women consulted during the menstrual period (38.7%)

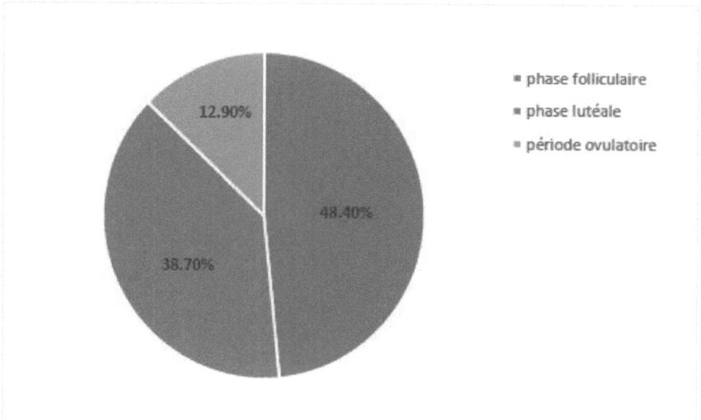

Figure 6. Phases of the menstrual cycle during patient consultations

2. Clinical study

2.1. Time between onset of symptoms and first medical consultation

This period varied from consultation within 12 hours of the first symptomatology to a period of more than 3 days.

Twenty-one patients (37.5% of cases) consulted within the first 12 hours.

Half of the patients (62.5%) were seen within 12 hours.

Nine patients consulted within more than 72 hours (Figure 7).

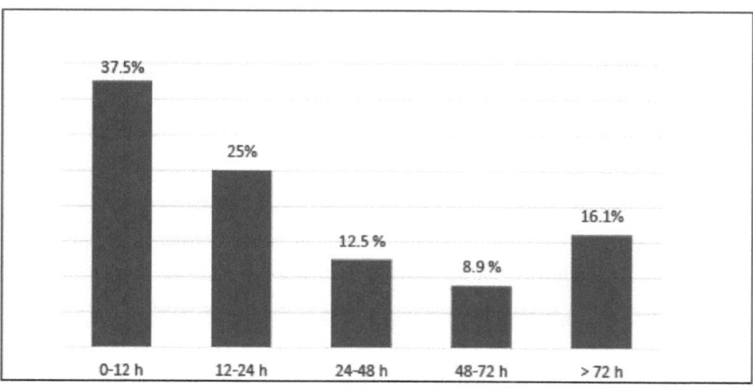

Figure 7. Time between onset of symptoms and visit to the gynaecological emergency department

2.2. Functional signs

2.2.1. Pain

Pelvic pain was the main complaint in 59 patients (98.3%).

- Mode of installation :

Pain was sudden in onset in 43 patients, or 71.7% of cases (Figure 8).

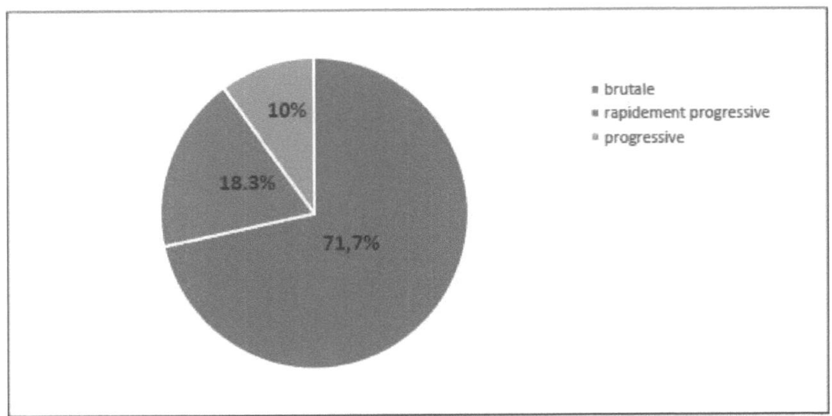

Figure 8. How pain develops

- Broadcast :

Pain was described as localised without diffusion in 45 patients, i.e. 75% of cases.

- Similar painful episodes :

Eight patients (13.3%) reported a similar episode of pain.

2.2.2. Associated signs

Digestive disorders such as vomiting were the most frequently associated sign in 41.7% of cases, followed by nausea in 6.7% of cases.

Urinary signs such as pollakiuria were only observed in two patients.

Only one case of associated metrorrhagia was noted.

3. Physical examination

3.1. General signs

General condition was considered to be unchanged in the majority of patients (81.7% of cases), whereas alteration of general condition with arterial hypotension was noted in 11 patients (18.3% of cases).

In our study series, 6 patients had a fever not exceeding 39°Celcius.

The other patients were apyretic.

3.2. Physical signs

3.2.1. Abdominal examination

- Location of pain :

Pain in the right iliac fossa was noted in 25 patients (42.4% of cases).

Pain in the left iliac fossa was noted in 19 patients (32.2% of cases).

Hypogastric pain was noted in 12 patients, or 20.3% of cases **(Figure 9).**

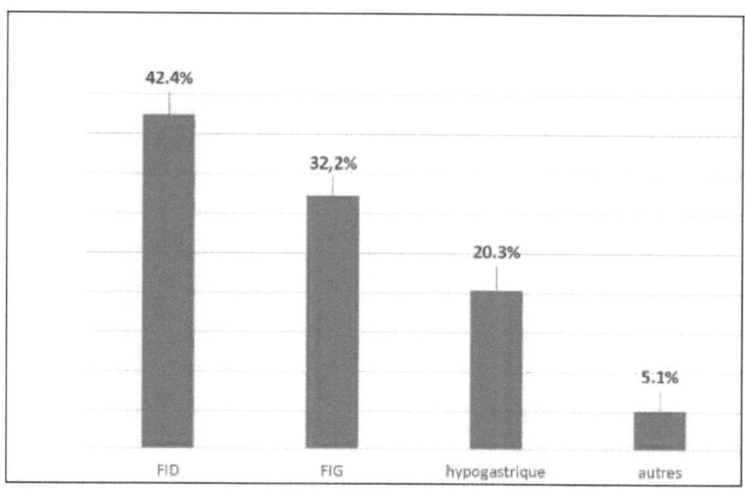

*Autres : inclus la douleur diffuse abdominopelvienne et lombaire

Figure 9. Location of pain during physical examination

- Intensity of pain :
- Pelvic sensitivity was found in 46 cases (76.7%).
- Pelvic tenderness was present in 14 cases (23.3%).

- Pain diffusion :

- Pain on palpation was localised in 48 women (80%).
- Pain spread to the rest of the abdomen was noted in the remaining 12 cases (20%).

3.2.2. Gynaecological examination

- Speculum examination was carried out in just one case and revealed a small amount of endo uterine bleeding.
- The vaginal touch was painful in 46% of the women examined.
- None of the patients had leucorrhoea.

-Table III shows a summary of the functional signs and physical examination findings in our patients (Table III).

Table III: Summary of the clinical study of patients

Clinical Study	Workforce	Percentage (%)
Functional signs :		
Pelvic pain	59	98,3
Sudden onset	43	71,7
Local pain	45	75
Similar painful episode	8	13,3
Nausees	4	6,7

Vomiting	25	41,7
Urinary signs	2	3,4
Metrorragies	1	1,7
Physical examination		
Change in general condition	11	18,3
Temperature (>38°)	6	10
Localisation of pain		
Right	25	42,4
Left	19	32,2
hypogastric	12	20,3
Abdominal defence	14	23,3

III. Paraclinical data

1. Blood count (CBC)

This examination was carried out in 53 cases, with WBC values ranging from 4200 elements/mm3 to 24700 elements/mm3. We noted hyperleukocytosis greater than 10000 elements/mm3 in 28 patients, i.e. 52.8% of cases.

2. C-Reactive Protein (CRP)

CRP levels were measured in 27 cases, and the threshold for positive CRP levels at our centre's laboratory is above 5 mg/L.

Thirteen cases (48.1%) had a positive CRP.

The CRP was 148.2 and 165.5 in two febrile patients.

3. Pelvic ultrasound :

Pelvic ultrasound was performed in all our patients.

The equipment used was that in the emergency room of our department, and 29 patients (48.3%) benefited from additional ultrasound examinations in the radiology department of the Monastir Maternity and Neonatology Centre.

Ultrasound scans were performed suprapubically in all patients, and 8 patients benefited from additional endovaginal ultrasound.

Pelvic ultrasound showed the presence of an adnexal mass in 49 women (81.7% of cases).

3.1. Topography of the mass :

The right-hand site was the predominant site, accounting for 43.6% of cases, followed by the left-hand site, which accounted for 34.5% of cases, and then the retrouterine, abdomino-pelvic, bilateral and supra-vesical sites (Figure 10).

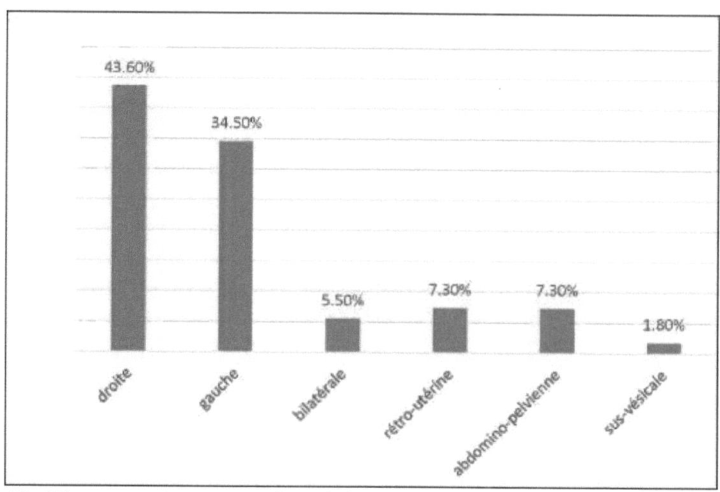

Figure 10. Ultrasound topography of the twisted adnexal mass

3.2. Dimensions of the mass

A study of the ultrasound size of the adnexal masses revealed an average size of 80.22± 3.6 mm, with extremes ranging from 3 cm to 20 cm.

Thirty patients, or 61.2% of cases, had an adnexal mass size of between 5 and 10 cm (Figure 11).

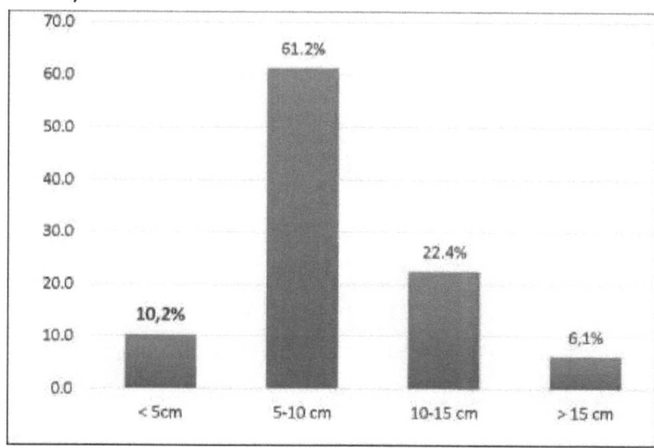

Figure 11. Distribution of ovarian masses by ultrasound size

3.3. Mass echostructure

The predominant sonographic appearance was anechoic in 41 cases (83.7%) (Figure 12).

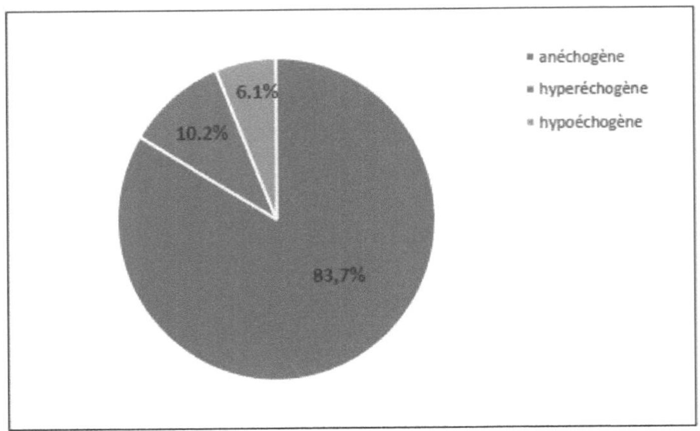

Figure 12. Echogenicity of the twisted adnexal mass

Solidocystic masses ët were found in 14 cases or 28%.

The typical ëchographic appearance of the dermoid cyst ë-was foundë in 3 women Eight cysts among the cysts ëtudiëes ëtaient cloisonnës soit 13,3 % et les vëgëtations ont ëtë dëcrites dans 4 cystes soit 6,7 % des cas (Tableau IV).

Table IV: Breakdown by content of adnexal masses

Echostructure	Workforce	Percentage (%)
Solid	5	10
Solid cystic	14	28
Heterogene	4	8
Appearance suggestive of dermoid cyst	3	6
Hemorrhagic	1	2

3.5. Ultrasound signs of torsion

The ëchographic signs of torsion ëtait notës in some reports d^chographie .

The ovary increased in size in 34 patients (56.7% of cases).

Hype^chogenic ovarian stroma ëtait notë in 5 patients or 8.5% of cases.

Peripheral arrangement of the follicles was noted in 7 patients, i.e. 11.7% of cases (Figure 13).

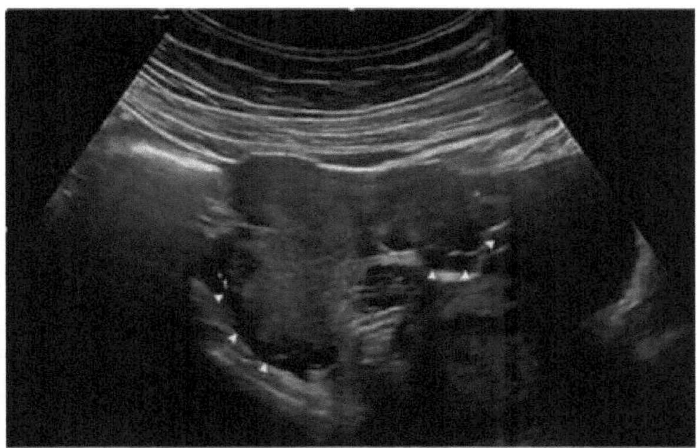

Figure 13. Enlarged ovary with peripheral arrangement of follicles (arrows) found by transabdominal ultrasound.

The Whirlpool sign was found in 7 patients, or 11.7% of cases (Figure 14).

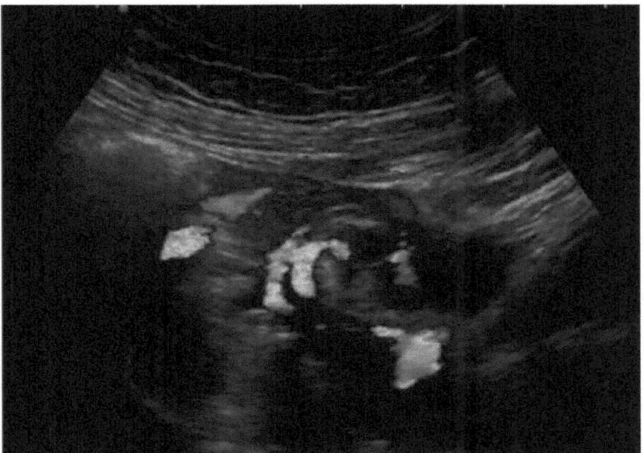

Figure 14. Whirlpool sign found by transabdominal colour Doppler ultrasound

3.6. Presence of effusion

Douglas effusion was present in 53.3% of cases (32 cases); it was judged to be of low abundance in 25 cases, i.e. a predominance of 80.6%, and of moderate abundance in the remaining 6 cases (19.4%).

No case was found where the effusion was considered to be very abundant.

4. Other additional tests

4.1. Abdominal and pelvic CT scan

Abdominopelvic CT scans were requested in 10 patients presenting with subacute forms or referred from general emergencies for suspected adnexal torsion discovered during this examination on suspicion of other pathologies.

Scannographic signs of torison were found in 5 cases:

- one ovary was increased in size in one case.
- abnormal position of the adnexa or adnexal mass in 3 cases.
- an image of the turn of the spire of the proboscis found in one case.

4.2. Pelvic MRI

No patients in our study series had pelvic MRI. Table V summarises the various biological and ultrasound data found in our patients during the diagnostic process (Table V).

Table V: Summary of para-clinical study of patients

Para-clinical study	Workforce	Percentage (%)
Biological data : Hyperleukocytosis (WBC>10000)	28	52,8
CRP > 5	13	48,1
Ultrasound data :		
Presence of adnexal mass	49	81,7
topography of the mass		
Right	24	43,6
Left	19	34,5
Medium size	8cm [3-30]	
Anechogenic mass	41	83,7
Ovary increases in size	34	56,7
Hyperechogenic ovarian stroma	5	8.5
Peripheral arrangement of follicles	7	11.7
Abnormal position of the adnexa/cyst	5	8.5
Doppler vascularisation of the adnexa		
Poorly vascularised	1	1.7
No vascularisation	5	8.5
Whirlpool sign	7	11.7
Twist sign	2	3.3
Douglas effusion	32	53,3

IV. Therapeutic attitudes

1. Time between consultation - admission to the gynaecology department and surgery

The average time from emergency consultation to surgery was 6.9 hours, with extremes ranging from 20 minutes to 38.5 hours.

The average time from admission to the gynaecology department to surgery was 3.6 hours, with extremes ranging from 10 minutes to 20.3 hours.

Four patients were initially admitted to the gynaecology department for clinical monitoring and reassessment, and when pelvic pain worsened, they were transferred to the operating theatre on suspicion of adnexal torsion.

2. Surgical exploration

2.1. Approach

Crelioscopy was performed in 37 patients (61.7% of cases).

Laparotomy for embolism was performed in 23 patients, i.e. 38.3% of cases.

2.2. Intraperitoneal effusion

Intraperitoneal effusion was noted in 26 women, i.e. 43.3% of cases, and was considered to be small in most cases, most often bloody or sometimes serous or lemon-yellow in colour.

2.3. Pathological appendix

- Torsion dimension :

We noted a predominance of adnexal torsion on the right side (58.2%).

There was one case of bilateral torsion in an 18-year-old girl (Figure 15).

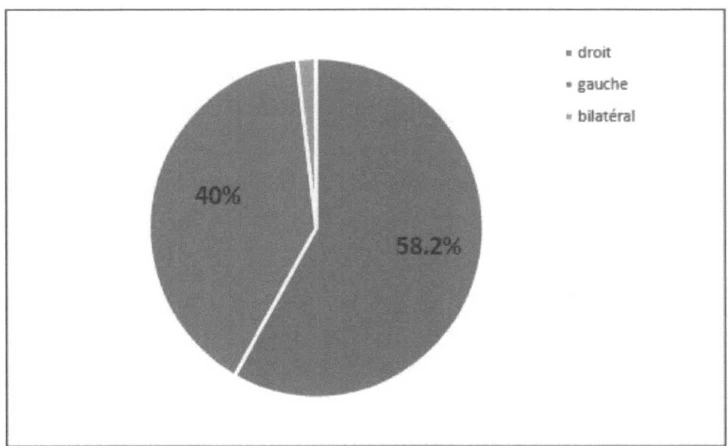

Figure 15. Dimension of the torsion in peroperatory

- Torsion on healthy or pathological adnexa :

Torsion on a pathological adnexa involved 50 cases:

- 49 cases of cyst torsion (81.6%)
- 1 case of tubal torsion on hydrosalpinx (1.7%)

Tubal torsion was diagnosed on suspicion of a 4 cm twisted cyst initially on suprapubic ultrasound in a 15 year old girl presenting with acute pelvic pain. A twisted hydrosalpinx and a healthy ovary on one side with a contralateral non-twisted cyst were then discovered intraoperatively.

Torsion on a healthy adnexa involved 10 cases of ovarian torsion (16.7%).

- Number of turns :

The number of turns of the coils varied from 1 turn to 6 turns in our patients, and in three operative reports the number of turns of the coils was not mentioned, including one case of a twisted 170 cm cyst where the number of turns of the coils was impossible to count because the cyst was fixed to the uterus with multiple adhesions (Table VI).

Table VI: Number of spiral turns observed

Number of turns	Workforce	Percentage (%)
1	14	24.6
2	19	33.3
3	15	26.3
4	6	10.5
5	2	3.5
6	1	1.8

- State of the twisted appendix :

The vitality of the twisted appendix was assessed after detorsion.

Thirty-eight adnexa had good vitality after detorsion (63.3%). Seven adnexa were of doubtful vitality (11.7%).

Fifteen adnexa, or 25% of cases, had a necrotic appearance on surgical exploration, ten of which regained colour after detorsion (Figure 16).

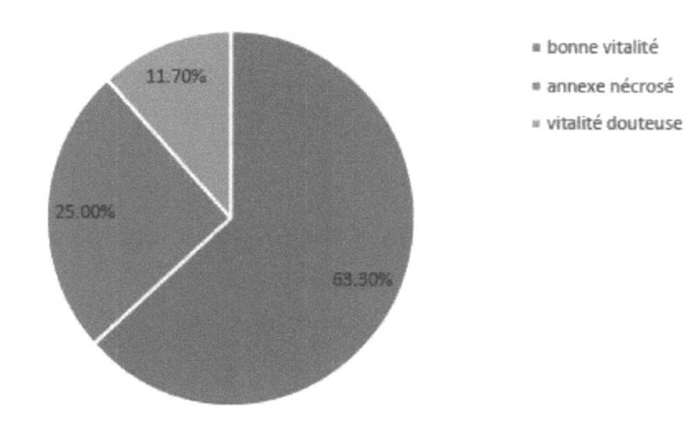

Figure 16. State of the twisted appendix during operative exploration

- associated adnexal pathology :

The presence of a cyst was confirmed in 49 cases, i.e. 81.6% of cases (Table VII).

Table VII: Summary description of adnexal pathologies associated with adnexal torsion

Adnexal pathology	Description	Percentage(%)
Seat of the ovarian cyst	44	89.7
Paratubal	5	10.2
Cyst size (cm) Mean	7	
Minimal	3	
Maximum	30	
Dermoid cyst contents	10	16.7
Endometriosis	1	1.7
Hemorrhagic	7	11.7
Lemon yellow	4	6.7
Serene	6	10
Sero-hematics	2	3.4

3. Annex controlateral

We have noted :

- five cases of non-twisted contralateral cysts.
- Most of the ovaries were normal except for one case of a tumoured ovary without associated torsion.
- The tube was abnormally long and tortuous in 8 cases, i.e. 13.6% At the end of this exploration, Table VIII summarises the different results found intraoperatively.

Table VIII: Summary of surgical exploration for adnexal torsion

	Workforce	Percentage(%)
Surgical approach :		
Colonoscopy	31	51,7
Laparotomy	23	38,30
Conversion	6	10
Blood effusion	26	43,3
Torsion dimension		
Law	37	58,2
Left	22	40
Bilateral	1	1.8
Healthy / pathological annex		
Healthy appendix	10	16.7
Pathological appendix	50	83.3
Number of turns	2,4 [1-6]	
Twisted appendix		
Good vitality	38	63.3

Questionable vitality	7	11.7
Appendix necrosis	15	25
Presence of adnexal mass	47	79,70
Average height(cm)	7 [3-30]	
Mass headquarters		
Ovarian	44	89,7
Paratubal	5	10,2

3. Treatment methods

3.1. Approach

Laparoscopy enabled treatment to be carried out in 31 patients, i.e. 51.7% of cases.

Laparoconversion was then performed in 6 patients because of operative difficulties.

Laparotomy for embolisation was performed in 23 patients, or 38.3% of cases.

3.2. Type of treatment

3.2.1. Conservative treatment

Conservative treatment was used in 52 patients, i.e. 86.7% of cases.

Detorsion alone was performed in 3 cases, combined with ovarian drilling in 3 cases and ovariopexy in 5 cases.

Detorsion with cystectomy was performed in 73.1% of cases (Table 12).

3.2.2. Radical treatment

It was performed on only 8 patients, or 13.3% of cases:

- Homolateral adnexectomy: 6 cases (10%)

. Five adnexectomies for necrotic sphacea of the adnexa

. Adnexectomy for suspected malignancy of the adnexa

- Bilateral adnexectomy: 2 cases of menopausal women (3.3%) All adnexectomies were performed by laparotomy.

Table IX summarises the different conservative and radical treatment modalities depending on the surgical approach chosen.

Table IX: Summary of the different conservative and radical therapeutic modalities depending on the approach.

	Laparoscopic approach (n=32)	Laparotomy (n=28)	Total (n=60)
Conservative treatment :			n=52
Detorsion	3	0	3
Detorsion + cystectomy	20	18	38
Detorsion + ovarian drilling	2	0	2
Detorsion +ovariopexy	3	1	4

Detorsion+ovariopexy+drilling ovarian	0	1	1
Puncture of cyst + detorsion	3	0	3
Tubal puncture + detorsion	1	0	1
Radical treatment:			n=8
Unilateral adnexectomy	0	6	6
Bilateral adnexectomy	0	2	2

3.3. Special cases

- Two women underwent tubal ligation, both aged 35 with a satisfactory number of children (>= 3), and the ligation was carried out after their written consent.
- A 42-year-old woman with a history of laparotomy cystectomy was found to have necrosis of the loop graft following occlusion on an associated flange. She underwent resection of the necrosis graft with ileostomy.
- For the 4 pregnant patients:
- Crelioscopy was the approach used for the 2 patients in the 1er trimester.
- Laparotomy was the chosen approach for the remaining 2 patients (2nd trimester).
- All these women had received intra-vaginal progestin treatment with antispasmodics.
- an associated tocolytic treatment based on a calcium channel blocker was prescribed for pregnant patients in the 2nd trimester (24SA and 26SA)

3.4. Intraoperative complications

We did not note any visceral or anaesthesia-related peroperative complications. However, we noted 9 cases of accidental cyst rupture during cystectomy (7 by crelioscopy and 2 by laparotomy).

V. Post-operative follow-up

1. Immediate

Immediate post-operative follow-up was straightforward in 58 women and complicated in 2:

- A woman presented with a urinary tract infection which progressed well under antibiotic treatment.
- One woman presented with a postoperative fever related to venitis and controlled by treatment with local LMWH. No thromboembolic or peritoneal complications were recorded in our series.

2. Post-operative stay

- The post-operative stay varied from 1 to 5 days.

- The average length of hospital stay after crelioscopy was 2 days, as was the length of hospital stay after laparotomy (Table X).

Table X: Length of hospital stay according to surgical route

Length of stay (days)	Laparoscopy	Laparotomy	Total
1	10	5	15
2	13	19	32
3	5	3	8
4	2	2	4
5	1	0	1
Total	31	29	60

- The average length of hospital stay after conservative treatment was 2 days, as was the length of hospital stay after radical treatment (Table XI).

Table XI: Length of hospital stay according to type of treatment

Length of stay (days)	Curator	Radical	
1	15	0	15
2	26	5	31
3	8	1	9
4	3	1	4
5	1	0	1
Total	53	7	60

3. Late Suites

3.1. Repeat offences

All our patients were reviewed postoperatively for control and anatomopathological results.

We noted 1 case of recurrence of adnexal torsion on a healthy homolateral adnexa after 1 year in a 13 year old girl who had undergone ovarian detorsion with ovariopexy.

3.2. Pregnancy progress

The 8-SA pregnancy was terminated at 12SA.

The 24-SA pregnancy was carried to term with an uneventful vaginal delivery.

The 2 other pregnant women were lost to view.

VI. Anatomopathological study

We obtained 43 histological reports of parts sent for anatomopathological examination.

1. Twisted appendix

Hemorrhagic infarction was the sign of histological necrosis described in 4 twisted adnexa (9.3%).

2. Twisted adnexal mass

Mature cystic teratoma was the most common histological type (28.6%) followed by serous cystadenoma (16.7%) (Table XII).

Table XII: Pathological findings in twisted adnexal masses

	Number	Percentage (%)
Corpus luteum cyst	5	11,9
Mature cystic teratoma	12	28,6
Serous cystadenoma	7	16,7
Endometriotic cyst	1	2,4
Mature teratoma + intestinal-type mucinous tumour	1	2,4
Follicular cyst	2	4,8
Benign ovarian cyst	5	11,9
Hydrosalpinx	1	2,4
Paratubal cyst	8	19
Necrosis of the appendix	4	9.3

3. Special cases

1er case : A mature cystic teratoma with a mucinous tumour of intestinal type with foci of invasive carcinoma was the only malignant tumour found in our series in a 23-year-old girl with no notable pathological antecedents who presented with paroxysmal hypogastric pain for 4 days with a huge solidolystic mass measuring 20cm on ultrasound and who had benefited from unilateral adnexectomy.

2eme case : A twisted endometriotic cyst with hemorrhagic necrosis of a graft loop following flange occlusion was found in a 43-year-old diabetic and hypertensive woman, G3P3A0, who presented with abrupt hypogastric pain with a 3 cm cyst associated with douglas effusion on ultrasound with no notable inflammatory syndrome on biology.

The patient underwent cystectomy with resection of the graft and ileostomy.

3eme cases: a right cystectomy with removal of the left ovary and removal of the peritoneum and epiploon was performed in a 34-year-old patient with no notable pathological history, G2P2A0, who was found to have a hypervascularised right ovarian tumour suspected of being malignant. The final anatomopathological result of the cystectomy performed was a serous cystadenoma of the right ovary with peritoneal and epiploic samples free of tumour proliferation.

4. Differential diagnosis

When the diagnosis of torsion was invalidated surgically, several other pathologies were found: hemorrhagic corpus luteum cyst in 13% of cases, followed by endometriotic cyst in 7% of cases.

Non-gynaecological causes included acute appendicitis in two cases (2%). In two other cases, no pathology was found (Table XIII).

Table XIII. Differential diagnoses found intraoperatively in cases of suspected adnexal torsion

Differential diagnosis	Numbers (n=40)	Percentage(%)
Bleeding corpus luteum cyst	13	13
Endometriotic cyst	7	7
Intracystic haemorrhage	2	2
Hemorrhagic ovulation	1	1
Other benign ovarian cysts*.	9	9
Acute appendicitis	2	2
Utero-annexal infection	4	4
Annexes : RAS	2	2

* includes serous cystadenoma, mucinous cystadenoma, follicular cyst and mature teratoma

VII. Analytical part

1. Prognostic factors for adnexal torsion

The analysis was based on the 60 cases of adnexal torsion surgically confirmed in our study. Five adnexa had a necrotic appearance at the time of surgical exploration, four of which were histologically confirmed. The results of the factors associated with adnexal necrosis are shown in Table XIV.

Larger cysts were significantly associated with necrosis (70 vs 150; p=0.05).

Table XIV: Predictive factors for necrosis of the adnexa

Factor	No necrosis(n=39)	Necrosis(n=4)	p
Age	26.9 ±9.6	31.5 ±5.06	0,354
Time between onset of pain and emergency consultation > 24h	11(30,6%)	1(33,3%)	1
Block_admission_deadline	3.3[1-3.5]	2.03[0.47-3.5]	0.749
T> 38°	4(10,5%)	0,00%	1
WBC>10000E/mm3	15(45,5%)	3(75%)	0,34
CRP>5 mg/L	7(46,7%)	1(50%)	1
Douglas effusion	17(43,6%)	2(50%)	1

Size of cyst(mm)	70[57-120]	150[80-220]	**0,05**
Cyst >5cm	35(94, 6%)	2(66, 7%)	0,214
Number of turns	2[1-3]	2[1,25-3,5]	0,751

2. Clinical-biological-radiological and operative comparison

2.1. Anamnestic factors related to adnexal torsion :

During the study period, 100 patients were admitted to the operating theatre with suspected adnexal torsion. The diagnosis of torsion was confirmed intraoperatively in 60 patients (60%).

The general characteristics of the two groups of patients with torsion (n=60) and without torsion (n=40) are shown in Table XV. The population in the torsion group had a younger mean age (25.92 ±9.09 vs 28.6 ±9.4), but this age difference was not significant (p=0.158). Nulliparous patients were present in 65% of cases in both groups. Torsion was significantly more frequent during the follicular phase of the cycle (75% vs 47.1%; p=0.045). The results of the remaining phases of the cycle (ovulatory period and luteal phase) were comparable with no significant difference. Antecedent cysts, cystectomy and adnexal torsion were similar in both groups. The notion of a similar painful episode was not significantly more frequent in the torsion group (13.3% in the torsion group vs 12.5% in the invalidated torsion group; p=0.903).

Table XV: Anamnestic factors associated with adnexal torsion

	No torsion (n=40)	Torsion (n=60)	P
Age (years)	28.6 ±9.4	25.92 ±9.09	0,158
Young girl	19 (47.5,9%)	37 (61.7%)	0,162
Gestite	0,5 [0-2]	0 [0-2,25]	0,946
Nulligest	23 (57.5%)	38 (63.3%)	0,558
Parite	0 [0-2]	0[0-0,75]	0,8
nulliparous	26 (65%)	39 (65%)	0,999
Phase of the menstrual cycle			
Follicular	5 (21.7%)	15 (48.4%)	**0,045**
Ovulatory	5 (21.7%)	4 (12.9%)	0,472
Luteale	13 (56.5%)	12 (38.7%)	0,194
Background			
Cyst	5 (12.5%)	8 (13.3%)	0,903
Cystectomy	4 (10%)	4 (6.7%)	0,710
Painful episodes	5 (12.5%)	8 (13.3%)	0,903

2.2. Clinico-biological factors associated with adnexal torsion

The clinical and biological data for the two groups are shown in Table II. Pelvic pain was the common clinical sign in both groups. There was no significant difference in the general and hemodynamic constants on admission: temperature, blood pressure and heart rate. Pain was generally described as located on the right side in both groups (43.5% vs 56.5%; p=0.512). Diffusion of pain was not significant in either group (20% for both groups). Abdominal guarding was rarely observed in both groups (17.5% vs 23.3%), with no significant difference (p=0.483). Vomiting was significantly associated with adnexal torsion in our series (20% vs 41.7%; p=0.024).

No biological factors were associated with the occurrence of torsion (**Table XVI**).

Table XVI: Clinico-biological factors associated with adnexal torsion

	No twisting (n=40)	Torsion (n=60)	P
General Signs : AEG	5 (12.5%)	11 (18.3%)	0,436
Temperature (°C)	37,1+0,43	37,14+0,42	0,896
Fever T > 38° C	2 (5.3%)	6 (10.2 %)	0.475
HR (bpm)	82,49+12,1	80,14+8,84	0,308
Localisation of pain			
FID	20 (50%)	25 (42.4%)	0,512
FIG	11 (27.5%)	19 (32.2%)	0,656
Hypogastric	7 (17.5%)	12 (20,3%)	0,755
Sudden onset	28 (70%)	43 (71.7%)	0.717
Abdominal defence	7 (17.5%)	14 (23.3%)	0,483
Diffuse pain	8 (20%)	12 (20%)	0,999
Associated signs : Nausea	5 (12.5%)	4 (6.7%)	0,478
Vomiting	8 (20%)	25 (41.7%)	**0,024**
Biological check-up			
CRP > 5 mg/l	12 (54.5%)	13 (48.1%)	0.656
Hyperleukocytosis (>10000)	19 (51.4%)	28 (52.8%)	0.89

2.3. Ultrasound factors associated with adnexal torsion

Where cysts were present, their median size was significantly greater in cases of torsion (p=0.004).

Torsion was significantly more common in cysts with anechogenic content (69.5% vs 34.8%; p=0.004) and significantly less common in cysts with hyperechogenic content (27.3% vs 10.2%; p=0.044) or heterogeneous content (25.8% vs 8%; p= 0.05). The presence of douglas effusion was not significantly associated with adnexal torsion (Table XVII).

Table XVII: Ultrasound factors associated with adnexal torsion

	No twisting (n=40)	Torsion (n=60)	P
Ovary increases in size	19 (47.5%)	34 (56.7%)	0,348
Hyperechogenic stroma	7 (17.5%)	5 (8.3%)	0.213
Peripheral layout of follicles	8 (20%)	7 (11.7%)	0.253
Abnormal position of appendix/cyst	4 (10%)	5(8.3%)	1
Presence of cyst	33 (82.5%)	49 (81.7%)	0,915
Location			
Law	19 (57.6 %)	24 (43.6%)	0,205
Left	13 (39.4%)	19 (34.5 %)	0,647
Size of cyst	60 [45,25-77,75]	82,5 [58,5-107,5]	**0,004**
Cyst > 5 cm	23 (67.6%)	44 (89.8%)	**0.012**
Content			
Solid	2 (6.5%)	5 (10%)	0,696
Cystic	13 (41.9%)	23 (46%)	0,5
Solid cystic	4 (12.9%)	14 (28%)	0,078
Heterogene	8 (25.8%)	4 (8%)	**0.05**
Echogenicite			
Anechogene	18 (54.5%)	41 (83.7%)	**0,004**
Hypo echogenic	6 (18.2%)	3 (6.1%)	0,147
Hyperechogenic	9 (27.3%)	5 (10.2%)	**0,044**
Reduced vascularisation / absent	3 (7.5%)	6 (10.2%)	0,738
Whirlpool Sign	3(7.5%)	7(11.9%)	0.736
Presence of effusion	20 (50%)	32 (53.3%)	0,744
Low abundance	15 (78.9%)	25 (80.6%)	0,999
Medium-large abundance	4 (21%)	6 (19.4%)	

2.4. Histological factors associated with adnexal torsion

Mature cystic teratomas and paratubal cysts were the two histological types significantly associated with adnexal torsion ((28.6% vs 3.8%; p=0.012) and (0% vs 8%; p=0.02) respectively, in contrast to hemorrhagic corpus luteum cysts and endometriotic cyst which were significantly more observed in the torsion-affected group (34.6% vs.

11.9%; p=0.024) and (23.1%vs2.4%; p=0.011) respectively.

Serous cystadenoma was observed in both groups without significant difference (Table XVIII).

Table XVIII: Histological factors associated with adnexal torsion

	No torsion(n=40)	Torsion(n=60)	P
Bleeding corpus luteum cyst	13(41.9%)	5(11.9%)	**0,003**
Serous cystadenoma	4 (15,4%)	7(16.7%)	1
Endometriotic cyst	7(22.6%)	1(2, 4%)	**0,009**
Teratomemature cystic	1(3.8%)	12(28.6%)	**0.012**
Paratubal cyst	0 (0%)	8(19%)	**0,02**

The factors significantly associated with torsion were :

- The follicular phase of the cycle
- Vomiting
- The presence of anechogenic cysts
- Cyst size > 5cm
- Mature cystic teratoma
- Paratubal cyst

4 DISCUSSION

I. Epidemiology

1. Frequency of twisting of appendages

Adnexal torsion is a rare cause of pelvic pain in women, ranking 5ème (12) with a frequency of 2 to 3% of all gynaecological emergencies in the paediatric population (20,21) and 2.7-7% in women of childbearing age (4) (6) (23).

The incidence of adnexal torsion is 6 per 100,000 women (24) according to a large study published in 2021, but the actual incidence of this condition in the general population remains poorly known because the definitive diagnosis is only made during surgery (4).

2. Age

Torsion of the adnexa occurs essentially during the period of female genital activity (25) (6) (26) (24). However, it can affect the extreme ages of life, ranging from the neonatal period (27) (28) to the postmenopausal period (29). In our series, the age of our patients varied from 13 to 53 years with a mean age of 25.92 ±9.09 years. Our results are consistent with those reported in the literature (Table XX).

Table XIX: Average age of patients diagnosed with adnexal torsion according to the literature

Author	Population (n=)	Average age
Ashwal (30) (2015)	208	27
Feng (31)(2017)	78	29,4
Melcer (1)(2018)	111	29,8
Resapu(32)(2019)	76	27
Moro(33) (2020)	315	30
Duan(34)(2021)	72	34
Our series (2022)	60	25,9

Melcer reported in his series of 199 cases of women admitted for suspected adnexal torsion that patients with adnexal torsion were significantly older than patients without torsion (29.8 ± 9.2 versus 26.8 ± 8.1 years, respectively, p=0.02). In our study, the mean ages of our patients were 28.6 ±9.4 for the non-torsion group and 25.92 ±9.09 for the confirmed torsion group with a p=0.158 so this difference was not significant. Our result is similar to that of Guven (35) and Gu (36).

3. Parite

Parity may play an indirect role in the determinism of torsion, according to Lee

Ch_(37) the strain placed on the abdominal wall by repeated pregnancies leads to relaxation and a certain atony of the abdominal muscles, thus favouring torsion. In the study by VijayalaKshmi (38) , 77.8% of patients had at least 2 children. On the other hand, Bardlin (11) noted in his series that the group of nulliparous women who presented 60.9% of all cases was significantly associated with adnexal torsion, contrary to Guven (35) who noted no significant difference (0.35±0.67 vs 0.15±0.34). For our series, no significant association was noted between nulliparity and the occurrence of adnexal torsion (Table XXI).

Table XX: Percentage of nulliparous women by series

Author	Population (n=)	Percentage(%)
Vijayalakshmi(2014) (38)	18	11,10
Resapu (2019) (32)	76	61,00
Bradin (2020) (11)	228	60,90
Meyer (2021) (39)	93	57
Our series	60	65

4. Phase of the menstrual cycle

Bharathi (40) observed that adnexal torsion occurred significantly during the post-ovulatory period and explained this phenomenon by pelvic venous congestion during this period which may be at the origin of the torsion. In his comparative study, Meyer (41) calculated the number of days since the last menstrual period and found a mean number of 21±21 for the confirmed torsion group and 21±13 for the confirmed torsion group, with no difference noted (p=0.924).

In our series, half of the patients (48.4%) consulted during the follicular period, its association with the occurrence of adnexal torsion was significant (p=0.045), this could be explained by the ovary increasing in size due to the increased size of the follicles during this phase and the evolution of the major follicle which could reach 3 cm and cause torsion.

5. Antecedents

5.1. History of adnexal pathology

5.1.1. History of ovarian cysts

Ovarian cyst is the adnexal pathology most incriminated in adnexal torsion (22) (25) (29). Ovarian cysts larger than 5 cm are known to be a risk factor for adnexal torsion (22) (25) (26) (42) (43) , However, torsion can occur with masses of any size, ranging from 1 cm to 30 cm according to Huang (25) (Table

XXII).

Table XXI : Frequency of antecedent ovarian cyst by series

Author	Population (n=)	Percentage(%)
Huchon (2012) (18)	29	58,60
Resapu (2019) (32)	76	71
Moro (2020) (33)	315	10,60
Our series (2022)	60	13,30

Huchon (44) noted in his comparative series that antecedent ovarian cyst was significantly associated with adnexal torsion (34 cases out of 142; p=0.04). In our series, no significant association between antecedent cyst and adnexal torsion was noted (p=0.903).

For previous cystectomy, the incidence of ovarian torsion varies from 2 to 15% in patients who have undergone surgical treatment of adnexal masses (25) (33). In our series, no significant association between antecedent cystectomy and the occurrence of adnexal torsion was noted (p=0.71).

5.1.2. Polycystic ovary syndrome :

Polycystic ovary syndrome has been identified as a risk factor for adnexal torsion (4) (26) (15). This condition has been implicated in 7% to 19% of cases of torsion(32) (45) . According to Warwar (42) , the weight of the extra ovary and the modification of its normal anatomy cause it to twist on its vascular pedicle, the lumbo-ovarian ligament. Individuals with polycystic ovaries have a non-modifiable risk of recurrence of torsion similar to the risk in children and adolescents, as the causative pathological mechanism also remains after simple detorsion (30). In a case series published by Brady (46), a 28-year-old woman with PCOS underwent unilateral ovarian torsion seven times over an eight-year period.

5.1.3. History of adnexal torsion

A history of adnexal torsion is considered by Ssi-Yan-Kai (15) to be the risk factor most associated with the occurrence of torsion. Recurrence can occur at any age (6) (Table XXIII).

Table XXII : Frequency of antecedent adnexal torsion by series

Author	Population (n=)	Percentage(%)
Ashwal (2015) (30)	208	29,80
Resapu (2019) (32)	83	22,90
Bardin (2020) (11)	76	3
Moro (2020) (33)	228	24,10

Meyer (2021) (39)	93	5.4
Meyer (2022) (41)	315	4,70
Our series (2022)	60	1.7

Dasgupta (47) reported in a review of the literature that the risk of recurrence of torsion in the paediatric population ranges from 5 to 18%. Possible explanations for the risk of recurrence include excessive mobility of the adnexa, venous congestion of the adnexa and abrupt body movements. According to Huang (25), the risk of recurrence may subsequently decrease as the ligament shortens when girls reach puberty.

Pansky (48) showed in a retrospective study that women who had a first episode of torsion with an ovary of normal morphological appearance were more likely to have another episode of torsion (60%) than those with a pathological adnexa (8%).

We have noted 1 case of recurrence of adnexal torsion on a healthy adnexa in our series after 1 year in a 13 year old girl who benefited from ovarian detorsion with ovariopexy.

5.1.4. Torsion of the adnexa and Medically Assisted Procreation (MAP)

Ovulation induction and ovarian hyperstimulation syndrome have been described as risk factors for adnexal torsion (26) (42) (43) (44). The risk of torsion associated with ovarian hyperstimulation syndrome increases further in pregnancy, from 2.3% to 16% in a retrospective study by Mashiach (4) of 201 stimulated cycles. Induction can result in multiple large ovarian follicular cysts which cause enlargement of the adnexa and thus carry an increased risk of torsion(15,25) (8).

In our series, a patient pregnant at 9 weeks' gestation after intrauterine artificial insemination (IAC) with her partner's sperm was admitted on suspicion of surgically confirmed adnexal torsion. She underwent intraoperative detorsion of her adnexa, which was found to be twisted without any associated adnexal pathology.

5.2. Previous tubal ligation

Tubal ligation may be a risk factor for adnexal torsion (22) (4) (15). It was incriminated in the genesis of torsion for the first time in 1952 by NOVAK (49). Damage to the mesosalpinx following electrocoagulation can lead to increased laxity of the tube resulting in torsion. In addition, the volume of the tube may be increased by tubal secretions preventing emptying into the uterus, resulting in hydrosalpinx (19172).

The rate of tubal sterilisation in series of women with ovarian torsion varies between 3.9% and 29% in the literature (22). Huchon (18) reported in his series that tubal ligation was not significantly associated with adnexal torsion. Asfour (22), on the other hand, in his review found that tubal ligation was a risk factor for subsequent adnexal torsion. In our series, two women (3.3%) had a history of tubal ligation.

5.3. Previous hysterectomy

Adnexal torsion can occur after interannexal hysterectomy, with a frequency of 3% according to the literature (17) (33).

Ogawa (29) has reported that torsion of a healthy adnexa is relatively frequent after laparoscopic hysterectomy and more often involves the right side. The subsequent increase in adnexal mobility and the lack of structural support for the uterus due to hysterectomy may contribute to torsion.

In our series, a single 40-year-old patient presented with adnexal torsion on a healthy adnexa and had previously undergone total inter-adnexal hysterectomy by laparotomy. She underwent ovariopexy with laparotomic ovarian drilling.

5.4. History of episodic pelvic pain

According to Moro (33) , 15.6% of patients reported a similar episode of pain. In Baron's series(50) , 30 women (38.5%) reported having had previous pain and 38 women (48.7%) had previously consulted a doctor for pain or an ovarian cyst. Sometimes, these episodes of pain can occur several days or months before admission, indicating an earlier partial torsion (26). The duration between these painful episodes varied from 1 to 210 days according to Huang's review (25). In our series, only 8 patients reported a similar previous episode, and similar episodes of pain were not significantly associated with subsequent torsion (p=0.903).

II. CLINICAL STUDY Clinical study

The clinical diagnosis of adnexal torsion remains difficult, not only because of the anatomo-clinical polymorphism but also because of the differential diagnoses with other gynaecological and surgical emergencies. However, the absence of pathognomonic signs should not obscure the value of good questioning and a thorough and meticulous clinical examination.

1. Clinical picture :

1.1. Functional signs

- Pelvic pain :

The most common symptom in women presenting with adnexal torsion is acute pelvic painë represented in 77.8% to 100% according to the literature(1,38) . The pain is due to occlusion of the vascular pedicle, with consequent hypoxia; in general, the venous and lymphatic systems are affected first because they are at lower pressure (4) , This pain may be described as constant or intermittent, as the ovary may twist and untwist over time and may twist with a sudden change in position or activity (4) (51) (Table XXIV) .

Table XXIII: Frequencies of acute pelvic pain reported as the main reason for consultation in the literature

Author	Population	Percentage(%)
Vijayalakshmi(2014) (38)	18	77,80
Nair (2014) (40)	70	95,70
Ashwal (2015) (30)	208	96,20
Melcer (2018) (1)	111	100
Wang (2019) (52)	174	79.82
Moro (2020) (33)	315	96,80
Our series (2022)	60	98.3

Pain is generally of abrupt onset, as described in the literature (18) (44,51) (2). In our series, it was noted in 71.7% of cases but this mode of onset was not significantly associated with adnexal torsion (p=0.71), unlike Huchon (44) who noted that abrupt onset and/or abrupt worsening of pain was significantly associated with adnexal torsion (p=0.03).

Pain during adnexal torsion is generally localized on one side only (18) (44) (4). In our series, pain was localised in 48 patients, i.e. 80% of cases, a finding similar to that of Ashwal (30) and Huchon (18) who noted that spontaneous unilateral pain was significantly associated with the diagnosis of adnexal torsion (p=0.0005).

Torsion occurs more frequently on the right, with an average frequency of 55 % according to the literature (53).this could probably be explained by the proximity of the left ovary to the sigmoid colon, which is relatively fixed, compared with the excessive mobility of the c^cum and ileum on the right (4,6,25).this explanation has also been found in the mechanism of torsion of healthy adnexa after hysterectomy according to Ogawa (29) (Table XXV).

Table XXIV: Frequency of right-sided pain in adnexal torsion, by series

Author	Population (n=)	Percentage(%)
Garner (2016)	302	62,90
Melcer(2018) (1)	111	55,90

Ghulmiyyah (2019) (10)	10	40
Moro (2020) (33)	315	60,30
Tzur(2021)(54)	19	47,40
Our series (2022)	60	42,40

Pain was found in 42.4% of cases on the right side in our series, with no significant difference when comparing this frequency with the confirmed torsion group, where pain on the right side was noted in 50% of cases (p=0.51). Our results are comparable to those of Melcer(1) who found no significant difference between the 2 confirmed and confirmed torsion groups (62/111 cases or (55.9%) vs 43/88 cases or 48.9%; p=0.6).

- Associated signs :

The signs generally associated with pelvic pain are nausea and vomiting explained by a vagal reflex secondary to intense pain (55) or by peritoneal irritation (33). In the literature, the frequency of these signs varies from 34.1% to 63.5% (30,34) but differs significantly according to age, with a marked incidence in the paediatric population (6).

For some authors (1,44,56), vomiting was considered to be a significant predictive sign of adnexal torsion, for others (53), (5),(11), vomiting was not a sign significantly associated with torsion and can be seen in various other digestive, urinary and gynaecological pathologies such as appendicitis, extrauterine pregnancy, colitis, necrosis of a leiomyoma and ruptured ovarian cysts (2,4). In our series, vomiting was significantly associated with adnexal torsion (20% vs 41.7%; p=0.024). Binary logistic regression analysis concluded that only vomiting was associated with adnexal torsion (OR= 0.35, CI95%=0.138-0.886).

Urinary signs, such as dysuria, although not specific (4), were present in 5.3% to 8.6% of cases (30) (38) (40), and in 3.3% of cases in our series.

Leucorrhoea and metrorrhagia were also rarely noted in adnexal torsion. In our series, only one patient out of 60 presented with metrorrhagia at the time of her emergency consultation.

Huchon (44) demonstrated in his prospective multicentre study that the presence of leucorrhoea or metrorrhagia made it possible to exclude low-risk patients without torsion (negative predictive value, 99.7%).

1.2. Physical examination

Because of its non-specific manifestations, the diagnosis of adnexal torsion may be difficult, which delays appropriate management and increases the likelihood of irreversible ischaemia and necrosis, making a thorough and meticulous physical examination essential.

- general signs :

The results of the general examination during adnexal torsion are generally non-specific (4). Fever was not a sign associated with torsion according to the literature, in fact its prevalence varies from 1.8 to 20% (1,2,9, 40, (38),43).In our study, the generally moderate fever of 38.5° was observed in 6 patients, i.e. 10.2% of cases, and was not significantly associated with necrosis of the adnexa (p=1). This finding is in line with that of Mazouni (57).

.

Tachycardia and high blood pressure are generally observed in cases of intense pain, but these characteristics are not significant in cases of adnexal torsion (4). In our series, general condition was maintained in 81.7% of cases and tachycardia was noted in only 4 patients (6.8% of cases).

- Physical signs :

Pelvic tenderness is found with a variable frequency ranging from 25.7% (40) to 84.1% (30). In our series, pelvic tenderness was noted in 76.7% of cases of torsion.

An abdomino-pelvic mass may be found on abdominal palpation, and is related to a cyst or an enlarged ovary (57). Its frequency varies in the literature from 9.8% (30) to 47% (43). Moore (4) demonstrated, in a retrospective study of 167 patients, that up to 75% of cases of proven adnexal torsion did not have a palpable mass. In our series, a mass was palpable in 2 cases (3.4% of cases).

The pelvic, vaginal and/or rectal touch can help to guide the examiner towards a genital pathology. Pelvic examination combined with abdominal palpation is often difficult because of the intense pain aroused by palpation of the cul de sac of the Douglas. This pain most often indicates peritoneal irritation (4) .

According to the literature, all these isolated or associated signs are not specific to adnexal torsion (53) (4) (57), apart from the exceptional "WAERNEK" sign cited by Horovitz (58), defined by the perception of a painful and palpable mass during pelvic examination corresponding to the twisted pedicle, and which is difficult to identify especially by rectal examination (58).

III. Additional examinations

1. Biological tests

To date, no biological marker has been found to confirm the diagnosis of adnexal torsion (35). Several markers of ischaemia, inflammation and infection have been the subject of several studies and clinical trials in an attempt to find a significant association between their levels and adnexal torsion. A beta hCG assay is imperative to rule out an extrauterine pregnancy (15).

1.1. Blood formula count

This is the only biological test that is consistently performed in emergencies. Most laboratory results are normal, although a slight leukocytosis may be observed in 20% to 63.3% of patients according to the literature (1,6,30,34,40,51), and hyperleukocytosis may be seen in the absence of fever (43). In our series, we noted a hyperleukocytosis greater than 10000 elements/mm3 in 28 patients, i.e. 52.8 % of cases, but this was not significantly associated with either adnexal torsion (p=0.89) or necrosis of a twisted adnexa (0.34). Our result is in contrast to that of Melcer (1) who noted that a hyperleukocytosis > 11000 elements/mm3 was significantly associated with adnexal torsion (p=0.01).

1.2. Proteine C Reactive :

This examination is not a routine examination, in fact, for our series, we found 12 cases or 20.4% where the CRP was judged positive, reaching 148.2 and 165.5 in 2 cases of febrile women, the elevation of the CRP was not significantly associated with adnexal torsion (6.15mg/l [2.2-31.85]; 3.55 [0.962-10.36] p=0.601). Our result is not in agreement with that of Huchon (44) who noted that a CRP<20mg/L was significantly associated with adnexal torsion (p=0.002) and that of Bakacak (59) who observed in his study that the CRP level was significantly higher in the adnexal torsion group (0.91 ± 0.18 vs. 0.39 ± 0.06 mg/l; p<0.001).

2. Radiological examinations

2.1. Pelvic ultrasound

Pelvic ultrasound is the first-line examination used to help diagnose adnexal torsion (10,11,13,60). It is relatively inexpensive, involves no exposure to ionising radiation and is widely available, but it is user dependent and may be difficult to perform in patients with significant pain (43).

Pelvic ultrasound has been used to diagnose adnexal torsion in 26% to 79% of cases in the literature (40) (14,43) with a sensitivity of 79% and a specificity of 76% according to the authors (60).

In our study, ultrasound scans were performed transabdominally in all our patients and 8 patients benefited from additional transvaginal ultrasound. The small number of transvaginal ultrasounds in our series is explained by the high frequency of young girls in our series (61.7% of cases).

2.1.1. Increased ovarian volume

Increased ovarian volume is the key ultrasound sign in the diagnosis of adnexal torsion (43,61,62). A volume difference of 5 ml between the pathological ovary and the normal ovary is considered significant by some authors (62). A twisted ovary may be rounded and enlarged compared with the contralateral ovary, due to redema or vascular and lymphatic congestion (25). (Figure 17).

An enlarged ovary was seen in 32.7 to 79.1% according to the series (6) (32,33) and with a mean size varying from 61 to 77 mm according to the literature. (6) (33) (30) . In our series, an enlarged ovary was noted in 56.7% of cases.

An enlarged redematous ovary was significantly associated with adnexal torsion (37.5% vs 80% ;p=0.03) according to the study of Ghulmiyyah (10). This result agrees with that of Melcer (1) and contradicts the findings of our series, in fact, this sign was not significantly associated with adnexal torsion (47.5% vs 56.7% ;p=0.348).

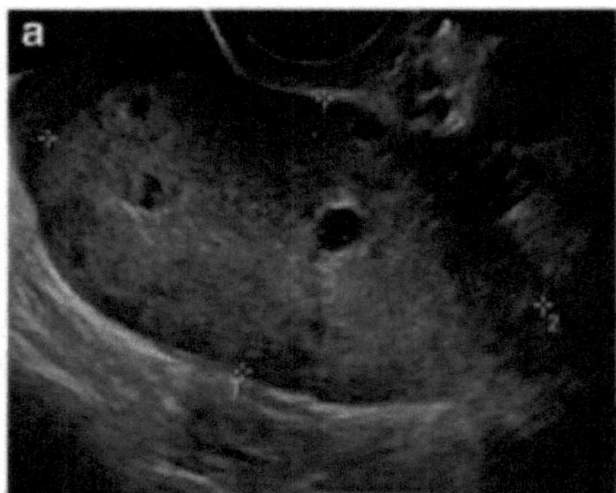

Figure 17. Torsion of the right ovary at the redematous stage in a woman of 44 years of age. Longitudinal ultrasound section showed an enlarged ovary measuring 7 cm in its largest dimension(61).

In a review of the recent literature published in March 2021, Strachovski (2) summarised five criteria which point towards ovarian enlargement during adnexal torsion (Figure 18).

Table 3: Manifestations of an Edematous Ovary at Imaging
Asymmetric enlargement (largest diameter >5 cm when no ovarian lesion is present)
Thicker than expected ovarian parenchyma surrounding a lesion
Peripheralization of follicles ("string of pearls" sign, "follicular ring" sign)
Free fluid adjacent to the ovary
Changes of parenchymal edema with or without hemorrhage (heterogeneity at US, increased attenuation at noncontrast CT, increased T1-weighted signal intensity at MRI)

Table 3: Manifestations of an Edematous Ovary at Imaging
Asymmetric enlargement (largest diameter >5 cm when no ovarian lesion is present)
Thidter than expected ovarian parendiym a surrounding a lesion
Peripheral nation of follicles ("string of pearls" sign.. "follicular ring" sign)
Free fluid adjacent to the ovary
Changes of parenchymal edema with or without hemorrhage (heterogeneity at US, increased attenuation at noncontrast CT. increasedTl - weighted signal intensity at MRI)

Figure 18. Radiological manifestations of an enlarged ovary according to Strachovski (2)

2.1.2. Hyperechogenic stroma :

Hyperechogenic stroma is the second ultrasound sign to look for, and may indicate a hemorrhagic infarct (43); its frequency in the literature varies from 2.4% to 25% (30) (57); in our series, hyperechogenic stroma was found in 8.5% of cases, with no significant difference from the surgically repaired torsion group (17.5%; p=0.213).

On ultrasound, stromal redema and hemorrhage may appear as hypoechogenic or heterogenous central areas (Figure 19).

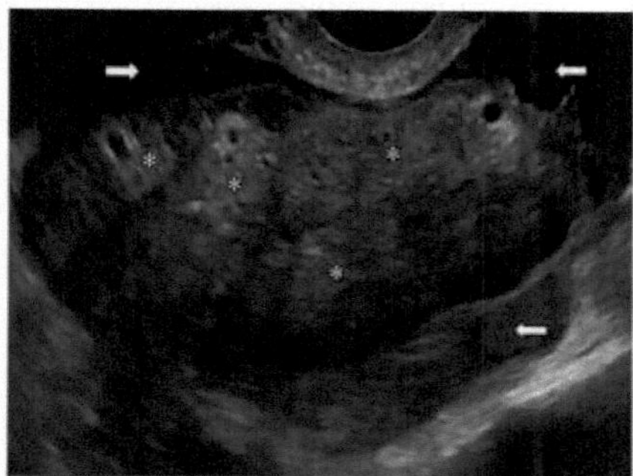

Figure 19. Transvaginal ultrasound image showing scattered focal hyperechogenicity (*), indicating a hemorrhagic infarct, which was confirmed

on histology (2).

2.1.3. Peripheral arrangement of follicles

In the case of torsion of the adnexa, the follicles may be arranged peripherally because they are pushed by the redeme of the ovarian stroma (53). According to Ssi-yan-kai (61) , an enlarged ovary with a central follicular stroma and multiple uniform peripheral follicles of 8-12 mm is associated with torsion in 74% of cases. The peripheral arrangement of follicles was found in 37% of cases in the Resapu study (32) and in 11.7% of cases in our series. There was no significant association between peripheral arrangement of follicles and adnexal torsion in our series (Figure 20).

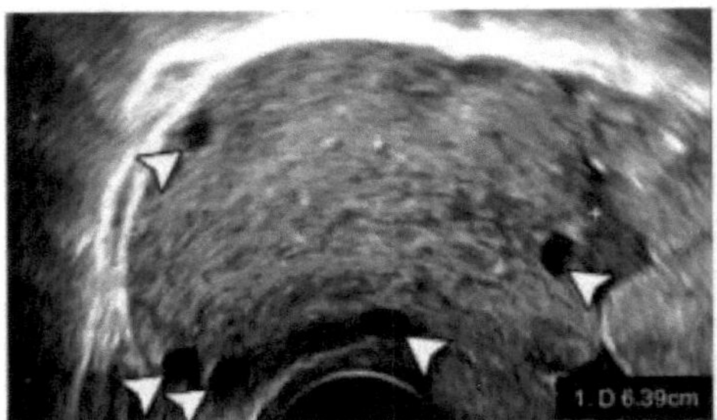

Figure 20. Transvaginal ultrasound image showing an enlarged ovary measuring 6.39 cm with peripheral hypoechogenic follicles (arrowheads) consistent with torsion(43).

2.1.4. Follicular ring sign

Another ultrasound finding is that of a hyperechogenic rim surrounding the peripherally displaced antral follicles, known as the "ring sign", with the rim measuring 1 to 2 mm thick. This sign is best seen by endovaginal ultrasound (43,61). Strachovski (2) reported that this appearance is due to engorged capillaries and haemorrhage in the thecal layer of the peripheral follicles. The follicular ring sign was noted in 38.1% of patients in Moro's series (33) and in 80% of patients in Sibal's study (63) (Figure 21). This sign was not mentioned in the ultrasound reports of our patients.

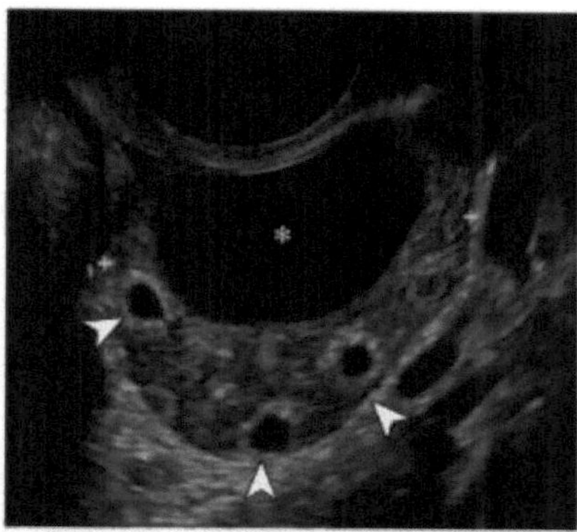

Figure 21. Transvaginal ultrasound image showing a 2.8 cm single ovarian cyst with increased echogenicity surrounding numerous follicles (arrowheads): Ring sign

2.1.5. Abnormal position of the adnexa / cyst

An inclination of the uterus or an unusual location of the ovary, very high or anterior to the uterus, very low or posterior to the uterus or median, are suspicious signs of torsion (2). This was noted in 34% of 315 cases of confirmed torsion according to Moro (33). Resapu(32) found an abnormal position of the adnexa in 54% of patients diagnosed with adnexal torsion. In our series, the adnexa had an abnormal position in 8.5% of cases and this sign was not significantly associated with adnexal torsion (p=1), unlike Ghulmiyyah (10) and Feng (31) who found that abnormal position of the ovary was significantly associated with adnexal torsion in their studies (Figure 22) (Figure 23).

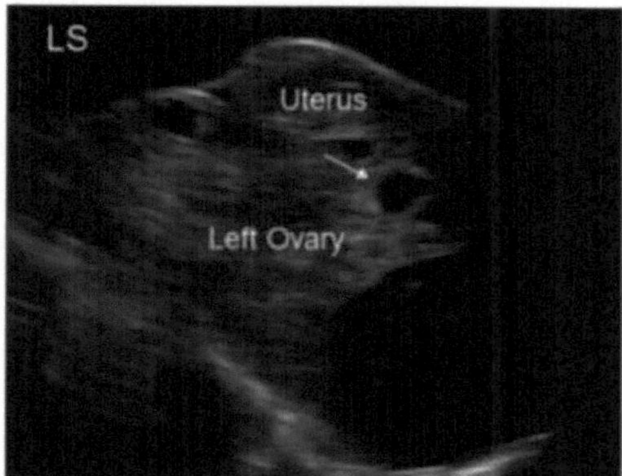

Figure 22. Twisted ovary enclosed in the cul-de-sac of Douglas, the uterus being in contact with the uterus.

forward (63).

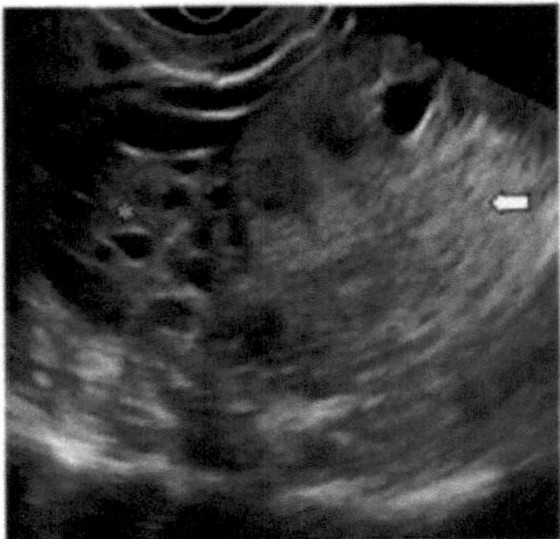

Figure 23 Transvaginal ultrasound of the right adnexa showing a normal right ovary (*) adjacent to a twisted and redematous left ovary (arrow) (2).

2.1.6. Presence of adnexal mass

Ultrasound can easily distinguish an ovarian mass by its echogenicity, location and content. The frequency of presence of an adnexal mass during adnexal torsion varies in the literature from 36% to 98.6% (40). In our series, 81.7% of our patients diagnosed with adnexal torsion had an adnexal mass on ultrasound, but this finding was not significant, our result is comparable with that of Ghulmiyyah (10) who did not note a significant association (40% vs 60%, p=0.3), these results contrast with those of Huchon (18) who found in his prospective study that the presence of a cyst on ultrasound was significantly associated with torsion with a sensitivity of 93.8% and a specificity of 53.6%.

In our series, we found that twisted cysts had a significantly larger mean size than the mean size of untwisted cysts Cyst size (60mm [45.25-77.75] vs 82.5mm [58.5-107.5] ;p=0.004), we also noted that cysts larger than 50mm were significantly associated with adnexal torsion, our result is consistent with the literature(22,25),(44). Bar-on (64) on the other hand found no correlation between the size of the adnexal mass and adnexal torsion in his series of 78 women admitted for suspected torsion.

Benign cysts are more likely to cause adnexal torsion (61) (22) , (4) . A complex ovarian mass on ultrasound was more frequently documented in menopausal patients (52.2% versus 25.4%, p<0.001), which may be explained by the fact that torsion involving malignant ovarian masses is rare (4) and because other symptoms usually dominate the presentation.

Ultrasound findings of dermoid cyst were significantly associated with torsion (p=0.02), whereas ultrasound findings of hemorrhagic corpus luteum cyst were more frequent in women without torsion in Melcer's study (1). Our anatomopathological results concur with these findings, in fact, after histological study, we found that dermoid cysts were significantly associated with adnexal torsion (1(3.8%) vs 12(28.6%); p=0.012).

In our series, torsion was significantly more common in cases of cysts with anechogenic content (69.5% vs 34.8% ; p=0.004) and significantly less common in cases of hyperechogenic cysts (27.3% vs 10.2% ;
p=0.044) or with heterogeneous contents (25.8% vs 8%; p=0.05). A detailed description of the echogenicity and contents is mandatory for any adnexal mass discovered on ultrasound (Figure 24).

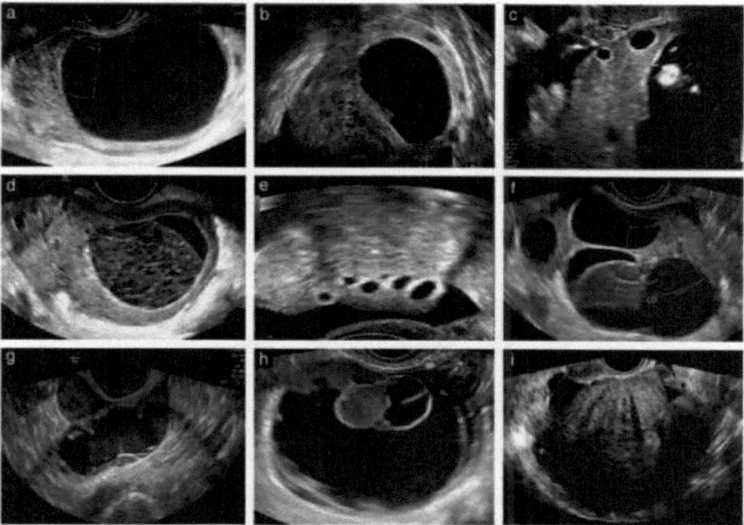

Figure 24. Ultrasound images of twisted ovaries with adnexal masses :

(a, b, f) serous cystadenoma; (c, e) mature cystic teratoma; (d) corpus luteum; (g) fallopian tube with pyosalpinx; (h) mucinous border tumour; and (i) fibroma. (33).

2.1.7. Douglas effusion

Although the presence of douglas effusion is seen in a variety of abdominopelvic diseases, a study of 47 positive cases by Dawood (43) showed that with ovarian enlargement, effusion is a sensitive sign of torsion. However, it is not specific and must therefore be correlated with the findings of the clinical examination and the other ultrasound signs. Its frequency in the literature is highly variable, ranging from 4.8% to 87% (30) (40) (2). The presence of effusion was significantly associated with adnexal torsion in the comparative studies by Feng (31) and Mashiach (14). In our study, Douglas-fir effusion was observed in 53.3% of cases, estimated in most situations to be of low abundance but with no significant association with adnexal torsion (p=0.744).

2.1.8. Doppler study

Doppler can be used to assess ovarian vascularity, although its usefulness in the diagnosis of adnexal torsion is controversial (43).

An abnormality of venous flow, defined as a non-continuous flow pattern, may be present in up to 100% of cases (43). Arterial flow may initially show a high impedance before becoming absent (4).

Studies have reported variable frequencies of abnormal colour Doppler flow in cases of torsion, ranging from 37% to 66% of cases (32) (40) (33).

In his recent review, Wattar(60) reported that the sensitivity of the Doppler study was 80% and that its sensitivity had a value of 88%. In his comparative study, Feng (31) noted that reduced or absent vascularity on Doppler was significantly associated with adnexal torsion (67 vs 10; p=0.03). In our series, 36 women had benefited from Doppler studies and decreased and/or absent vascularity was noted in 6 patients in the confirmed torsion group, i.e. 10.5% of cases, with no significant association with torsion (p=0.73) (Figure 25).

It is important to note that normal Doppler studies should not be used to exclude torsion or delay surgery in the presence of a high index of clinical suspicion(2). Indeed, Moro found in his study of 315 patients with confirmed torsion that half (56%) had preserved vascularity on Doppler.

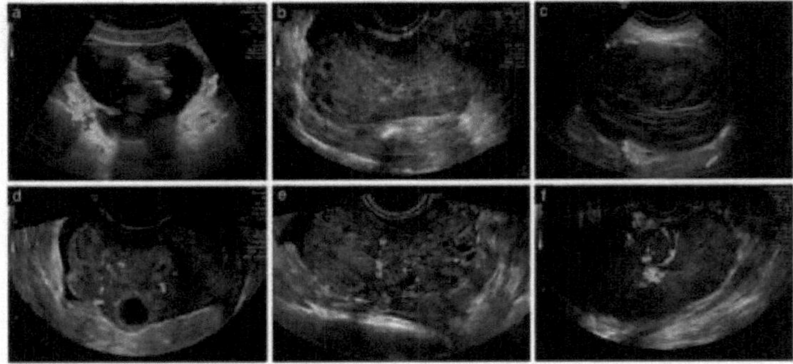

Figure 25. Colour Doppler ultrasound images of twisted ovaries with no vascularisation (a-c) and preserved vascularisation (d-f)

- The Whirlpool Sign

In a recent review, Dawood (43) reported that Doppler study can help to appreciate the swirling vessels in the twisted pedicle or "swirl sign". Transvaginal ultrasound facilitates dynamic assessment in several planes to identify this sign, which will be termed the "target" sign (concentric alternation of hypo- and hyperechogenic rings) if visualised perpendicular to the axis of rotation (2) (Figure 26).

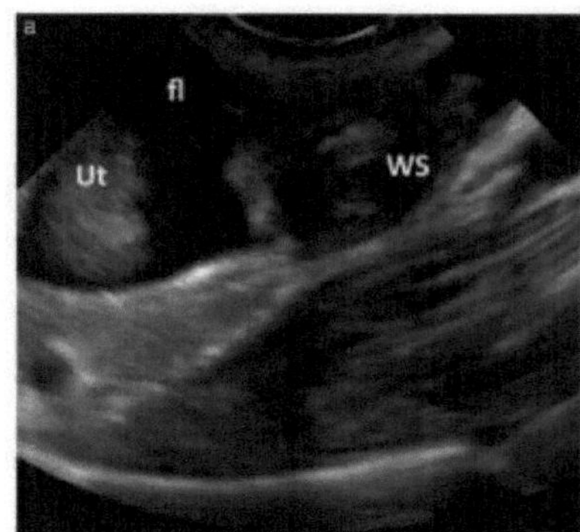

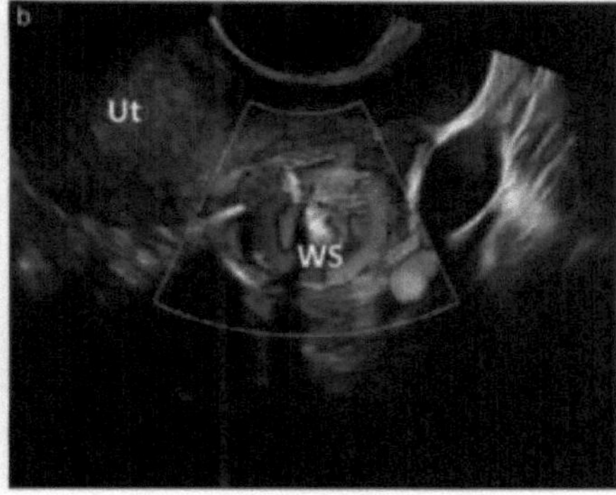

Figure 26. Colour Doppler ultrasound image of the whirlpool sign. ut: uterus; fl: effusion; ws: whirlpool sign. (65).

Several authors have reported a high sensitivity of the Whirlpool sign for the diagnosis of adnexal torsion ranging from 90.8% to 98% (31,33) (11,65). In our series, Whirlpool's sign was seen in 7 patients (11.9% of cases) but was not significantly associated with adnexal torsion (p=0.736).

The presence of a swirl sign is not always a confirmatory sign of adnexal torsion, in fact, Feng (31) noted that 40% of women suspected of having adnexal torsion who were confirmed intraoperatively, had a swirl sign on ultrasound. In our series, the swirl sign was seen in three patients in the group with torsion that had been invalidated.

2.2. Computed tomography

Although CT is not indicated in cases of suspected torsion, it is often performed in women presenting with acute non-specific abdominal pain(43). The common CT findings of adnexal torsion according to the authors (61,66,67) are displacement of the adnexa towards the contralateral side or in the median position (68), deviation of the uterus towards the side of the ovary concerned, enlargement of the adnexa, thickening of the wall of the suspected mass (67) and the presence of swirl signs (69)(Figure 28).

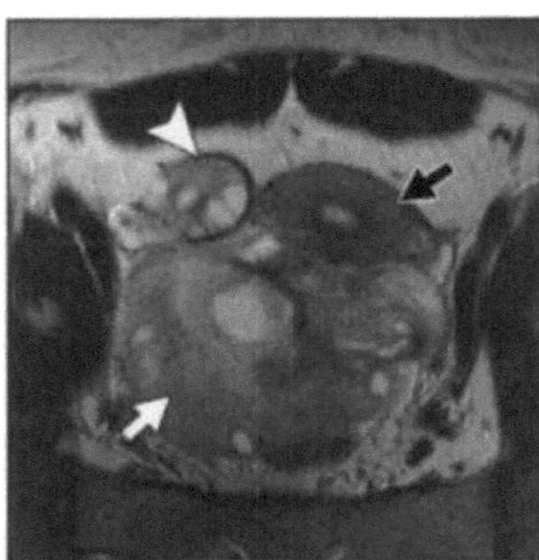

Figure 27. The uterus (black arrow) is deviated to the left by the enlarged and twisted left ovary (white arrow). The normal right ovary is visible (white arrow)(70).

Duan (34) in his recent series published in 2021 evaluated the feasibility of preoperative prediction of torsion angle by CT to stratify the risk of necrosis in patients with adnexal torsion and found that the risk of adnexal necrosis is high in patients with a torsion angle >720°. An enlarged twisted pedicle and pedicle hemorrhage are CT findings that can be used to predict a torsion angle >720 and may indirectly imply adnexal necrosis (Figure 29).

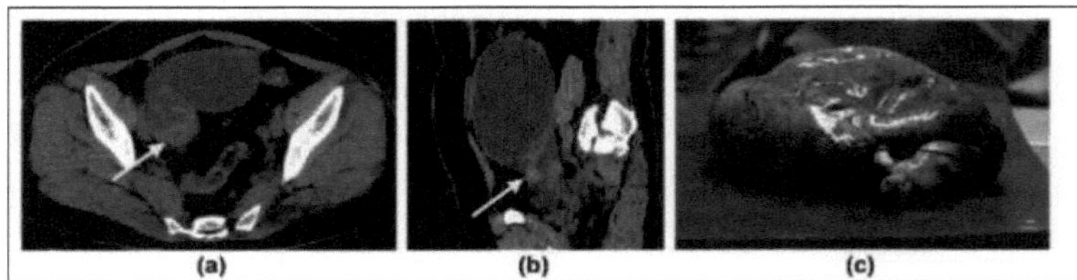

Figure 28. Axial CT image showing the cyst with an enlarged twisted pedicle (a). Punctiform haemorrhage visible at the margin of the torsion pedicle. (Sagittal reconstruction images showing the twisted pedicle with hemorrhage (arrows, mass sign) (b) Photograph of the piece showing the necrotic ovarian tissue and the twisted pedicle: a torsion angle of 1.080° was noted (c) (34).

Bronstein(13) and Swenson (71) reported in their comparative studies that the performance of ultrasound and CT for the diagnosis of adnexal torsion was similar.

In our series, CT scans were performed in 14 patients, i.e. 14.1% of cases. The small number of cases in which CT evidence of torsion was found did not allow us to carry out an analytical study of these results. It is also important to note that a tumoured adnexa with peripheral arrangement of follicles was found in 2 women without torsion being found intraoperatively.

3. Magnetic resonance imaging

Magnetic resonance imaging (MRI) is expensive but useful for diagnosing ovarian torsion if ultrasound findings are equivocal or in pregnant women (53). MRI offers a better soft tissue study and can demonstrate the components of a complex ovarian mass in greater detail than ultrasound (60). However, delays caused by additional diagnostic studies may make MRI inadvisable (61).

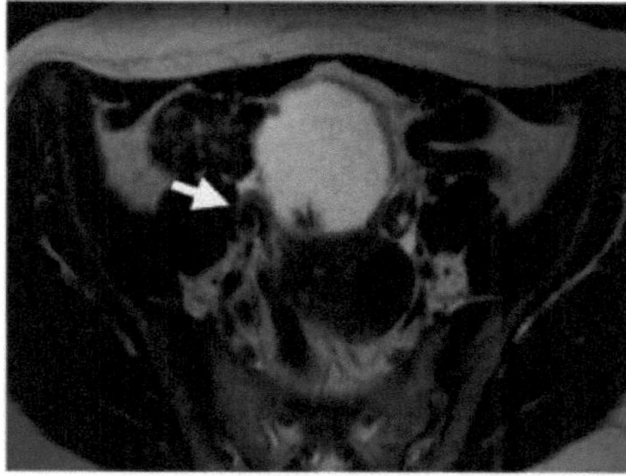

Figure 29 .T2-weighted transverse MRI image shows the whorl sign. A twisted right fallopian tube (arrow) is seen in a 57 year old woman with subacute pain.

IV. CLINICAL FORMS Clinical forms

1. Subacute and chronic symptoms

According to the literature, subacute torsionë is defined by pain lasting no more than 2 days and chronic torsion is defined by pain lasting more than 3 days (72) . These forms are less frequent (72).

The symptoms are fleeting and paroxysmal, sometimes giving way spontaneously (73), most often explained by episodes of torsion-detorsion of the adnexa, lasting from a few days to several months (53). Questioning is therefore a precious and vital part of the diagnosis. The physical examination is not very specific and may reveal a latero-uterine adnexal mass with varying degrees of pain on palpation. Takeda (72) found in his series that women presenting with chronic torsion were significantly older and that half of these women were admitted for planned adnexectomy with discovery of a twisted adnexa intraoperatively.

2. Topographical shapes

2.1. Isolated torsion of the fallopian tube

Isolated torsion of the fallopian tube is a rare event (74) To date, the reported incidence of fallopian tube torsion in the literature is 1:500,000 to 1:1,500,000 (75). Isolated torsion of the fallopian tube may occur as a result of extrinsic masses such as ovarian and paratubal cysts (53), intraperitoneal adhesions, pregnancy (76) and pelvic congestion (74) or intrinsic causes which are hydrosalpinx, hematosalpinx, abnormal mesosalpinx length (15) and tubal ligation (74). A large number of case reports, case series and reviews about fallopian tube torsion involve paediatric and adolescent patients (5,54,75,77,78), suggesting that tube torsion may be more common in young people.

The clinical signs of torsion of the tube are not specific, and are most often represented by acute pelvic pain with a possible adnexal mass on physical examination (79).

The typical appearance of tubal torsion on ultrasound is that of a dilated, redematched tube with thickened echogenic walls (74) . The dilated tube may be found in the middle of a normal homolateral ovary, narrowing towards either end in a configuration known as the "beak" sign (43),(53).The ultrasound swirl sign is the specific sign of tubal torsion, but it is not always fully detectable, especially in the presence of a mass.(15)

In our series, an isolated torsion of the tube was noted in a 15 year old girl who presented with severe pelvic pain in the context of apyrexia with an enlarged ovary and a 4cm cyst on ultrasound with the discovery of a twisted hydrosalpinx with a contralateral non-twisted cyst intraoperatively. The patient benefited from tubal puncture followed by detorsion of the tube with laparoscopic cystectomy.

Given that the majority of patients are adolescents (5,53,75), tubal preservation should be preferred wherever possible, due to concerns about future fertility (80).

2.2. Para-ovarian and paratubal cysts

Paratubal cysts are remnants of the mesonephric (Wolffian) ducts (2). They are simple benign cysts separated from the ovary (81) which are often attached by a peduncle to the mesosalpinx (2) and account for 10% of all adnexal masses (81). According to the literature, they are usually complicated by haemorrhage and rupture, but rarely by torsion (81). These cysts may twist on their own or predispose to isolated tubal torsion (5).

The diagnosis of paratubal cyst torsion can be difficult, as patients present with signs and symptoms of ovarian torsion but normal-appearing ovaries on imaging (2). Imaging findings in the literature include a median cystic mass and beak or swirl sign adjacent to the torsed structure (74).In our series, we noted 8 paratubal cysts, but the initial clinical examination of all patients was similar to the examination of patients admitted for ovarian cyst torsion so it can be concluded that knowledge of this phenomenon and particular attention to extraovarian structures are essential to the diagnosis (2,12).

2.3. Bilateral torsion

This is an exceptional situation which may occur simultaneously (82) or more often successively (83-85). This situation is certainly rare (86) and the clinical picture is very misleading, but it should always be considered in the presence of a patient who has already undergone surgery for this condition or in the presence of a patient presenting with diffuse pelvic pain and more than one cystic mass on ultrasound (86,87). In our series, we observed a case of simultaneous bilateral torsion in an 18 year old girl who presented with acute pelvic pain with vomiting that had been evolving for one day, with two cystic masses measuring 60 and 85 cm on ultrasound, with visualization of a Doppler turn of spire on the right side. The patient benefited from detorsion of the two adnexa with bilateral cystectomy of the two paratubal cysts by laparotomy.

2.4. Torsion on healthy appendix

Normal-appearing ovaries are involved in up to 46% of cases of torsion (4). This condition can occur at any age, however, particularly in prepubertal girls with elongated lumbo-ovarian ligaments (25) and in pregnant women (88). The clinical picture is unremarkable.

Ultrasound remains the reference examination, enabling differential diagnoses to be eliminated and indirect signs of ischaemia to be sought. Interruption of venous flow leads to a reactive remodelling which can be detected by the increase in ovarian volume compared with the contralateral adnexa (88). The usefulness of ovarian vessel Doppler remains controversial (89). MRI is a satisfactory complementary investigation technique in pregnant women, with greater accuracy than ultrasound. The combination of Doppler and MRI provides a better diagnostic approach, but should not delay surgical management(88).

In our series, we observed 10 cases of isolated ovarian torsion without associated adnexal mass, i.e. 16.7% of cases.

3. Forms according to age of onset

3.1. Antenatal torsion

This is an exceptional form. The first case was published in 1961 by Karrer and Swensen (90) . There are not many cases reported in the literature. The clinical picture may mimic or cause acute intestinal obstruction in neonates (91,92) and radiological suspicion is often raised antenatally by the discovery of an abdominal cystic mass in the fretus (93). In 2020, Saeed (94) published the case of a neonate in whom a complex solid avascular mass was observed on antenatal ultrasound. The operation was performed after 5 weeks of life and an ovarian necrosis was discovered. Treatment was oophorectomy. Kurtmen (93) published in 2021 a series of 28 newborns in whom an abdominal cystic mass was diagnosed antenatally and which corresponded to a twisted ovarian mass at laparoscopy, in 61.7% of cases, auto-amputation of the ovary was noted. All cases were treated by oophorectomy.

3.2. Torsion in children and adolescents

Adnexal torsion is the fifth most common gynaecological emergency and accounts for 2.7% of all cases of children with acute abdominal pain (51). Unlike in the adult population, torsion of a healthy adnexa can occur in up to 25% of cases in the paediatric population due to physiological elongation of the lumbo-ovarian ligament, excessive mobility of the fallopian tube or abrupt body movements (vigorous exercise, sudden changes in body position, increase in intra-abdominal pressure, trauma)(25) (47) .

Careful questioning can be a valuable diagnostic tool if it reveals similar episodes or a sudden onset of symptoms. However, vomiting was significantly associated with adnexal torsion according to the recent study in 2021 by Tzur (54) and Ashwal (30). The clinical diagnosis is completed by a transabdominal ultrasound scan, which may find an enlarged ovary associated with a cystic image, most often benign in appearance (41,53). Abdominopelvic CT and MRI scans should be requested if there is any doubt about the diagnosis and should never delay surgical management in order to preserve subsequent fertility in children and adolescents (3).

3.3. Torsion and pregnancy

Adnexal torsion during pregnancy is a rare nosological entity (95) . It represents 2.7% of all surgical emergencies in pregnant women (96). Its incidence varies from 3 to 5 per 10000 pregnancies. Pregnancies induced by MAP techniques are the most likely to be complicated by torsion (97,98) (4). This complication is more frequently encountered during the 1er trimester (88,96,99,100), more rarely during the 2me trimester (89,101) or the 3me trimester (76,102). In our series, 2 women presented in the 1er trimester (8 and 9 SA) and 2 women in the 2nd trimester (24 and 26 SA). No cases were noted during the 3me trimester of pregnancy in our series.

During pregnancy, there is an increase in the volume of the gravid uterus, resulting in elongation of the suspensory ligaments of the ovary, the ovarian fringe and the uteroovarian ligament, associated with physiological uterine dextrorotation, which leads to uncoupling and separation of the various adnexal elements from their origins (89). These changes make the adnexa more vulnerable to torsion in the presence of pre-existing adnexal pathology (88) but torsion in a healthy adnexa is not uncommon during pregnancy (76,101). Pregnancy is therefore considered by most authors to be a risk factor for adnexal torsion (4,25,39).

Adnexal masses that cause torsion during pregnancy are generally between 6 and 8 cm in size (4), and are usually presented by corpus luteum cysts and dermoid cysts (99,102). MRI without gadolinium contrast is often used when the source of pain cannot be identified using ultrasound(25).In our series, all pregnant women benefited solely from transabdominal ultrasound, which alone enabled the diagnosis of adnexal torsion to be suspected.

3.4. Post-menopausal women

Adnexal torsion is a rare cause of pelvic pain in menopausal women, as the associated signs are vague and the diagnosis of torsion is rarely made (104). Cohen (7) noted in his comparative study that fever was significantly more marked in postmenopausal women diagnosed with adnexal torsion than in premenopausal women. This may be explained by the long delay between the first symptoms and their consultation, which could lead to necrosis of the adnexa and subsequent continuous dull pain and fever. The delay in surgery in menopausal women may be explained by misdiagnosis and additional pre-surgical work-up for pelvic masses with a higher suspicion of malignancy and a reduced suspicion of torsion in these patients.

In our series of adnexal torsion, 2 women were menopausal and underwent bilateral adnexectomy. Pathological examination of the 2 adnexa revealed two twisted ovaries with two serous cystadenomas of the ovary. Bilateral adnexectomy is no longer the treatment of choice for such cases, in fact in recent years the treatment of adnexal torsion has been evaluated, and the majority of authors currently recommend unilateral adnexectomy (7,105) (106).

VI. Factors in delayed diagnosis

Early diagnosis of adnexal torsion is the only guarantee of conservative treatment. Although the development of ultrasound and crelioscopy has made a major contribution to improving the management of adnexal torsion, diagnosis remains difficult in a number of cases. This difficulty may lengthen the diagnosis time, which is a determining factor in conservative treatment (9,50).

1. Factors inherent to the patient : Delayed consultation

The time between the onset of painful symptoms and the visit to the emergency department is a prognostic factor for the vitality of the appendix. Several authors have studied this time (Table XXVIII.).

Table XXV: Time between onset of symptoms and emergency department visit in the literature

Author	Year	Average duration
Nair(40)	2014	5.4 days (2-14)
Ganer (20)	2016	26.7 hours +/-33.7 hours
Wang(52)	2019	62.6 hours
Duan(34)	2021	54.5 hours
Hageg(75)	2021	8.75 hours

Ashwal (30) found in his study that the consultation time for impubertal girls was significantly longer than that for women of childbearing age. This was explained by the fact that only two-thirds of impubertal patients underwent pelvic ultrasound and 12% were not initially seen by gynaecologists.

In our series, it was impossible to calculate this exact time because only 8 patients out of 60 specified the exact time of onset of pain before their emergency consultation. For all our patients, this approximate time was estimated on the basis of the date of onset of pain and the date and time of the emergency consultation, which varied from a consultation within 12 hours of the first symptomatology to a time of more than 3 days. Contrary to the results of the literature (1,57), we did not find a significant association between the duration of consultation > 24 hours and necrosis of the adnexa (p=0.187).

2. Factors related to symptomatology

These are the most decisive factors for the clinician, represented by the subacute and chronic forms whose symptomatology is vague and misleading. For this reason, thorough questioning, a meticulous clinical examination and targeted radiological examinations seem necessary to support the diagnosis. In our series, subacute forms presented in 21.4% of cases and chronic forms in 16.1%.

3. Factors inherent in medical management

The time elapsed between consultation in the emergency department and transfer to the operating theatre for exploration and treatment is considered by some to be a determining factor in the prognosis of a twisted adnexa (9).

Table XXVI: Time between consultation at the gynaecological emergency department and transfer to the operating theatre

Author	Year	Timeframe (hours)
Nair (40)	2014	24
Glanc (9)	2015	22,4
Cohen (7)	2017	15
Wang (99)	2020	14
Hageg (75)	2021	5,45
Our series	2022	6,9

The apparent delay in carrying out the laparoscopy once the decision had been taken was explained by the patients' refusal to undergo an emergency operation during the night, the need to stabilise patients suffering from additional systemic diseases, and the anaesthetist's request for a full 6 hours.

It should be noted that many authorities consider that a short delay of a few hours is not detrimental to the future viability of the ovary(9) (50).

V. Differential diagnosis

The clinical diagnosis of adnexal torsion is difficult not only because of the clinical polymorphism but also because of the non-specificity of biological and radiological examinations. Several studies, such as our study, included in their series any woman who consulted for acute pelvic pain with suspected adnexal torsion on the basis of clinical and radiological examination data. Confirmation or denial of torsion was followed by surgery. The accuracy of 60% in the preoperative diagnosis of adnexal torsion in our department was comparable with previous studies reporting rates ranging from 44%-78%. (50,56,107)

Table XXX illustrates some of the studies published in the literature, with results divided into confirmed and rejected torsion groups.

Table XXVII. Clinical and operative comparison of women presenting with adnexal torsion according to the literature

Study	Twist	No twisting	Total	Study period

Zangue (2016)(108)	67	217	284	feb. 2013-dec 2014
Melcer (2018)(1)	88	111	199	jan2008-dec2014
Baron(2010)(50)	36	42	78	nov2006-feb2008
Huchon(2012)(18)	31	465	496	sept2006-avril2008
Guven (2015) (35)	24	14	34	3 years
Gu 2018 (36)	46	61	96	march2012-nov2017
Feng (2017) (31)	109	86	195	janv2020-june2015
Bardin(2020) (11)	270	52	322	1010-2016
Michelis (2021) (107)	42	6	54	january2009-july2014
Meyer (2022) (41)	83	37	121	march2011-june 2020
Our study (2022)	60	40	100	jan2017-janv2022

The diagnoses found during surgical exploration are of surgical and gynaecological origin (4) .

1. Gynecological causes

1.1. Extra uterine pregnancy

It may be diagnosed in the presence of a favourable background and amenorrhoea associated with pelvic pain. Confusion with adnexal torsion may arise when a hematosalpinx mimicking an adnexal mass is seen on ultrasound. A negative Beta-hCG assay formally rules out the diagnosis. However, the association of adnexal torsion with extra uterine pregnancy is possible, and cases have been published in the literature (109,110). In our series, all the patients were admitted to the operating theatre after verification of Beta HCG negativity, apart from the 4 cases of women known to be pregnant.

1.2. Utero-annexal infection

It may simulate adnexal torsion in the presence of a painful mass in a febrile setting. On ultrasound, tubo-ovarian abscess presents as a complex latero-uterine mass with septa, a thick tubal and/or ovarian wall and heterogeneous echogenicity. Vascular flow is strongly increased on Doppler. MRI provides the best assessment of the diffuse pelvic mass with debris, thickened septa and high contrast (15). Sendy (111) published in 2020 the case of a 23 year old patient who presented to emergency with severe pelvic pain and a complex right cystic image with preserved Doppler vascularisation. Laparoscopy revealed a bilateral pyosalpinx treated by bilateral salpingotomy.

In our series, we found 3 cases of tubo-ovarian abscess and one case of hydrosalpinx on surgical exploration. The 4 patients were apyretic but had a positive CRP ranging from 26 to 45 with hyperleukocytosis reaching 22240 in one patient. It can be seen that the presence of a biological inflammatory syndrome is an important factor that must be taken into account when discussing the diagnosis of adnexal torsion.

1.3. Intracystic haemorrhage

The clinical diagnosis between adnexal torsion and intracystic haemorrhage is often difficult, especially as these two complications may occur together. Haemorrhage may occur in a follicular cyst or, more commonly, in the corpus luteum cyst. On ultrasound, a rounded hypoechogenic avascular image with a meshwork or fine reticular pattern is found (112). There are typically multiple fine strands of fibrin giving a net-like appearance (15). Haemorrhagic cysts may resemble solid or solidocystic masses, due to the formation of blood clots and thicker septa within the cyst. Patients with hemorrhagic cysts larger than 5cm are usually followed up at 6-8 week intervals to demonstrate resolution or reduction in size in order to exclude the possibility of a bleeding ovarian tumour(15).

In our study, hemorrhagic corpus luteum cyst was the most common differential diagnosis with a frequency of 13%, followed by intracystic hemorrhage in 2 cases (without histological precision of the type of cyst) and hemorrhagic ovulation in 1 case. However, the association of hemorrhagic cyst with torsion is possible. In our series, five twisted cysts were hemorrhagic corpora lutea.

1.4. Torsion of a uterine fibroid

She is interested in the myoma under the serous pedicle. Questioning reveals the history of a fibroid that is already known. Ultrasound is the key examination because it can differentiate a liquid image from a fibroid with denser echogenic juxta-uterine content (113). In any case, surgical exploration is indicated in the presence of intense pain. In our series, we found a case of torsion of a pedicle uterine fibroid in a 14-year-old girl who presented with intense pelvic pain without associated fever. Ultrasound revealed a 47 mm anechogenic image. Laparoscopic exploration revealed a hemorrhagic corpus luteum cyst and a twisted uterine fibroid. A cystectomy and resection of the fibroid were performed. Follow-up was straightforward.

1.5. Ovarian hyperstimulation syndrome

This syndrome is generally seen in women undergoing medicated ovarian stimulation (112) . It generally occurs during the luteal phase or at the start of pregnancy. Clinical signs other than abdominopelvic pain and vomiting may include oliguria and dyspnoea due to pleural effusion (114) . The ovaries are enlarged with multiple cysts, sometimes reaching 25 cm. An untwisted hyperstimulated ovary has cysts separated by septa of thin tissue and is relatively symmetrical in size to the opposite side (15).

1.6. Uncomplicated adnexal pathology

This entity is found in 7% to 44.1% of cases in series {1_,2). It represented 16% of cases in our series, mainly endometriomas and cystadenomas of the ovary.
Ultrasound signs of torsion were present in five ultrasound reports, such as increased ovarian volume (n=5), peripheral arrangement of follicles (n=4), hyperechogenic stroma (n=4) and presence of Whirlpool sign (n=3), whereas operative findings showed normal-looking ovaries with uncomplicated adnexal pathology, This may be explained by the clinician's fear of missing a torsion, and therefore his decision to explore even if there was no strong clinical suspicion of a diagnosis of torsion, and by the influence of this clinician on the radiologist's request for additional ultrasound to confirm the suspicion of a diagnosis of torsion.

2. Non-gynaecological causes

2.1. Acute appendicitis

This is the first diagnosis to be made in the presence of acute pain in the right iliac fossa. The diagnosis is all the more difficult if the torsion occurs in a healthy adnexa. study of the appendix must be carried out systematically at the same time as ultrasound evaluation of the right ovary if adnexal torsion is suspected(15). If there is any doubt about the diagnosis, crelioscopy should be performed.
In our series, acute appendicitis was found in two women admitted for suspected adnexal torsion, the first of whom was apyretic, presenting with left iliac fossa pain with hyperleukocytosis and a CRP of 23.9 on biology and the presence of a 47mm cyst with an enlarged ovary on ultrasound, it is likely that the location of the pain did not prompt the clinician to consider the diagnosis of appendicitis of usually right location. In the second patient, the pain was on the right in a context of apyrexia with a CRP of 59 and normal WBCs. A 40 mm cyst on the right was seen on ultrasound with an enlarged ovary, a peripheral arrangement of follicles and a hyperechogenic stroma, hence the decision to explore by crelioscopy.

2.2. Others :

Other rarer diagnoses are possible, such as nephritic colic, acute urine retention, pelvic thrombophlebitis or diverticulitis.
Table 35 shows the frequency of differential diagnoses found by the authors.

(Table XXXI)

Table XXVIII.Differential diagnoses found intraoperatively in women presenting with adnexal torsion

Author	Extra-uterine pregnancy	Utero-adnexal infection	Intracystic haemorrhage	Appendicitis	Uncomplicated ovarian cyst	Other
Baron (2010) (64)	–	–	10,20%	–	29.5%	adhesions-PCOS
Huchon (2012) (18)	30,10%	14,80%	16,10%	1,20%		necrobiose fibroids- SHO-urological causes
Guven (2015) (35)			32,30%	8,80%		*■■■■
Zangue (2016) (108)	8,40%	1,16%	7,60%	9,35%	7%	
Feng (2017) (31)	1%	2%	1%	1%	4,61%	cystic rupture
Melcer (2018) (1)			26,60%		9,50%	Leiomyoma
Otjen (2020) (28)		1,50%	5,10%	5,40%	3,60%	urological causes - gastroenteritis
Bardin (2020) (11)		8,80%	47%	5,80%	44,10%	
Our series (2022)		4%	16%	2%	16%	

V. Recommendations

The diagnosis of adnexal torsion remains a challenge for all gynaecologists, given the clinical polymorphism and the sometimes inconclusive biological and radiological data.

In the future, prospective randomised clinical trials analysing a larger number of cases should be carried out to determine more precise diagnostic criteria and optimal treatment. This will improve the management of women with adnexal torsion. Conservative treatment by laparoscopy should be the treatment of choice whenever possible (8,106).

In the light of our findings and the review of the literature we have studied, we recommend :

- Raising awareness of this condition among emergency doctors.

- Bringing together the various clinical, biological and radiological semiological elements in the diagnosis of acute pelvic pain
- The need for a systematic gynaecological examination combined with pelvic ultrasound in any woman presenting with acute pelvic pain
- Doppler flow alone should not guide clinical decision-making
- Emergency laparoscopy in cases of suspected adnexal torsion
- The use of crelioscopy should be extended to cases where there is diagnostic doubt about another gynaecological or surgical emergency.

The following decision algorithm is also proposed for suspected adnexal torsion (Figure 32) and acute pelvic pain (Figure 33).

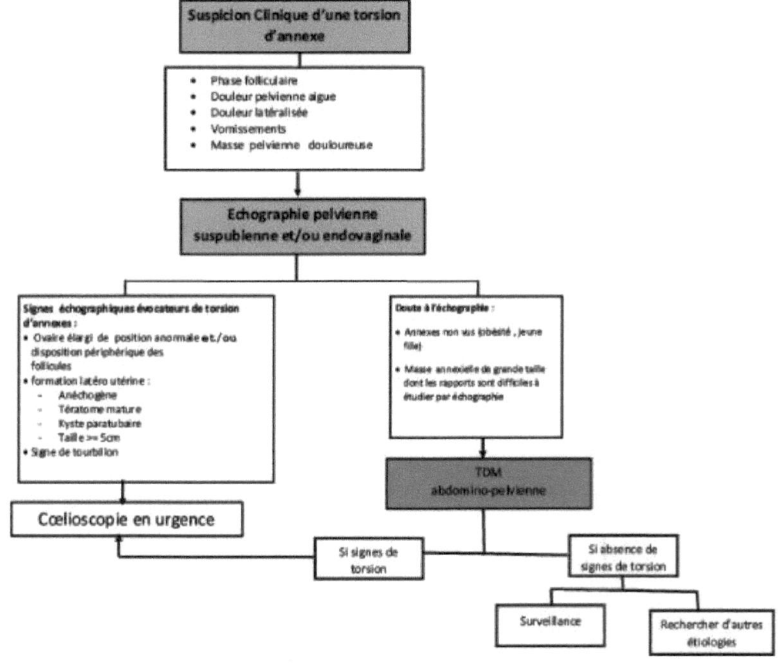

Figure 30. Decision-making algorithm for suspected adnexal torsion

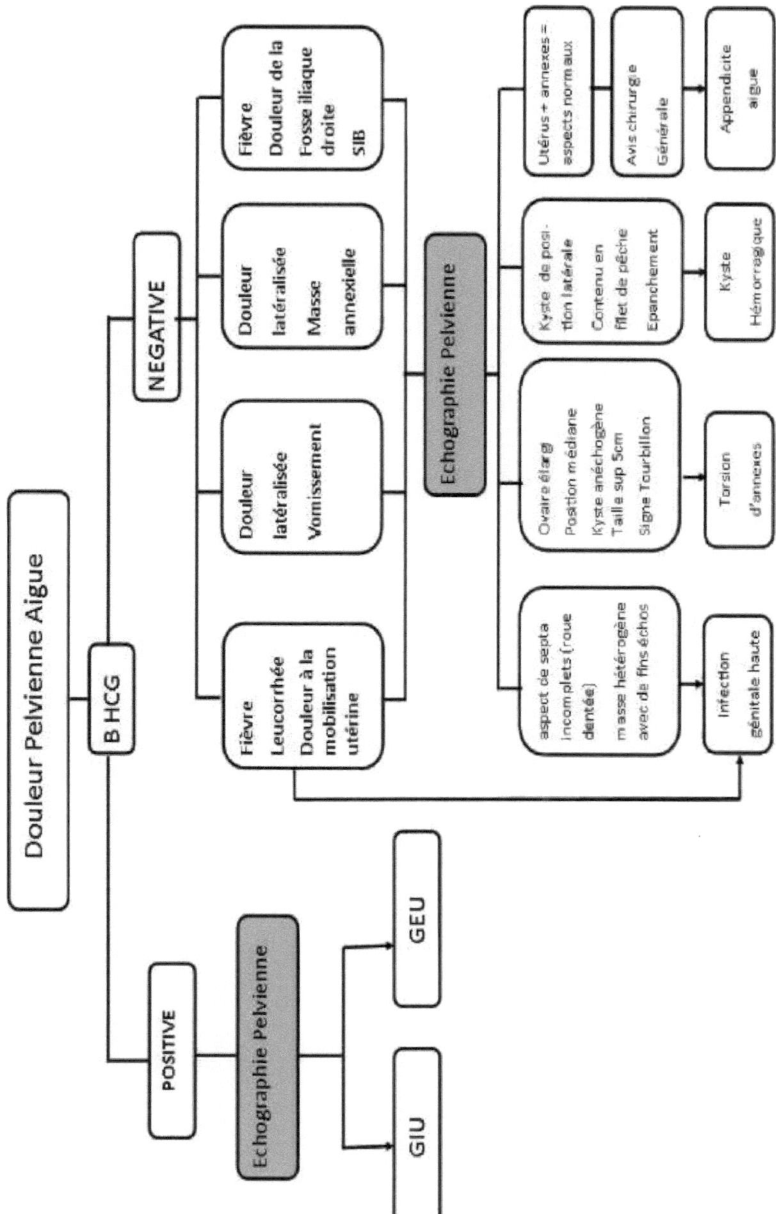

Figure 31. Decision-making algorithm for acute pelvic pain

VI. Limitations of the study

-Our study is limited by its retrospective design in data analysis. We were unable to obtain information on the severity of patients' pain, which could be associated with adnexal torsion.

-We also noted a lack of information in the files about cervical examinations carried out on female patients.

-Information on ultrasound results is based on a retrospective review of ultrasound reports and reflects the operator's subjective impression of the majority of ultrasound parameters studied.

-Most ultrasound scans were performed suprapubically, whereas optimal study of the adnexa should be performed transvaginally. The high frequency of virgin girls in our series may explain this limitation.

-Our series included only a small number of studies of ultrasound signs of torsion such as peripheral arrangement of follicles, hyperechogenic stroma and abnormal position of the adnexa, as well as a small number of Doppler flow studies.

-Our study was also limited by its monocentric nature. It would be interesting to conduct a larger, or even multicentre, study on a national scale to better describe and codify the clinical, biological and radiological signs associated with adnexal torsion, and to propose a composite score to help clinicians strengthen their diagnostic suspicion of adnexal torsion.

VII. Highlights

- Our study is the first nationwide study to look for a significant association of different clinical, biological and radiological signs with adnexal torsion.
- the use of these combined criteria may allow patients to be triaged for urgent surgery when the suspicion of adnexal torsion is high, as opposed to admission for observation and reassessment when the suspicion of adnexal torsion is low.

5 CONCLUSION

adnexal torsion is a surgical gynaecological emergency, its pathogenesis is multifactorial and remains poorly elucidated, but it seems that the keystone of all these mechanisms is the existence of an adnexal mass.

A retrospective study of 60 cases of patients admitted for torsion of the adnexa at the Gynecology-Obstetrics Department of Monastir from 1[er] January 2017 to 31 January 2022 showed that this pathology represents 14.93% of all gynecological emergencies.

Epidemiologically, this condition can be seen at any age, with an average age of 25.92±9.09 years and extremes ranging from 13 to 53 years, and a predominance of young women of childbearing age (93%). Young girls represented 63% of the total study population and 39 patients were nulliparous at the time of diagnosis (65%).

In our series, we noted 4 cases of pregnancy associated with torsion of the adnexa: two cases of pregnancy in the 1st trimester, one of which was induced by CAI, and two cases of spontaneous pregnancy at 24 and 26 days' gestation.

The majority of women consulted during the ovulatory period of the menstrual cycle, and we found that this phase of the menstrual cycle was significantly associated with the occurrence of adnexal torsion.

At the clinical stage, 37.5% of our patients consulted within 12 hours of the onset of pain, and the majority (62.5%) consulted after 12 hours. In fact, adnexal torsion can present as two main clinical pictures:

- an acute picture dominated by pelvic pain, found in 98.3% of our patients, with a sudden onset, unilateral, generally right (42.4%), violent, and possibly associated with digestive signs. Vomiting, found in 41.7% of cases, was significantly associated with torsion. Fever, not exceeding 39°C, was noted in only 6 patients (10.2% of cases) and was not significantly associated with adnexal torsion or necrosis.
- The "sub-acute" and "chronic" pictures are rarer, occurring in 16.1% of cases, where the pain is atypical, lingering, not very intense, and may date back a few days or even months. Spontaneous subtorsion or torsion-detorsion phenomena may explain these pictures.

The role of biological tests in the diagnosis of adnexal torsion is limited. CRP >5 mg/L and hyperleukocytosis were not significantly associated with adnexal torsion.

Pelvic ultrasound is an essential means of supporting the diagnosis of pelvic syndrome in women. All our patients underwent preoperative ultrasound, which revealed an adnexal mass in 81.7% of cases and an enlarged ovary in 56.7% of cases. Masses with anechoic contents, larger than 5 cm, seen in 89.8% and 83.7% of cases respectively, were significantly associated with adnexal torsion. In contrast, cysts with hyperechogenic or heterogeneous contents were significantly associated with the surgically reversed torsion group. The performance of ultrasound for the diagnosis of adnexal torsion is limited when it is performed trans-bdominally or when the radiologist is influenced by the clinician's diagnostic suspicion. In fact, ultrasound signs of torsion such as ovarian enlargement with peripheral arrangement of the follicles were found in reports of other diagnoses made intraoperatively.

Colour Doppler is an indisputable aid not only to positive diagnosis by demonstrating a reduction in vascular flow at the level of the ovarian pedicle and the presence of a vascular whirlpool sign found in 11.9% of cases in our patients, but also in 3 patients in the disabled torsion group.

From a diagnostic point of view, the anatomical and clinical polymorphism of torsion sometimes makes diagnosis difficult, and often poses the problem of differential diagnosis with other gynaecological and surgical emergencies, which will be resolved by surgical exploration. In fact, once the diagnosis of torsion is suspected on the basis of clinical arguments, with severe acute pain dominating the picture, and on the presence of an adnexal mass on clinical examination and/or ultrasound. Crelioscopy must be performed as a matter of urgency. It is used to confirm the torsion, to determine the severity of the adnexal lesions and, if necessary, to ensure treatment.

In our series, for every 100 women admitted urgently to the operating theatre with suspected adnexal torsion, the diagnosis was confirmed in 60 patients (60% of cases). Crelioscopy enabled the diagnosis to be made in 61.7% of cases and treatment to be carried out in 51.7% of cases. Conservative treatment of twisted adnexa was the treatment of choice in 86.7% of cases, reflecting our particular concern for preserving the adnexa and subsequently the fertility of our patients. Adnexectomy was performed for severely necrotic or sphacelic adnexa or for suspected malignancy. The two menopausal women had also undergone bilateral adnexectomy. Malignant tumour was found in only one case in our series. This was a mature cystic teratoma with an intestinal-type mucinous tumour with foci of invasive carcinoma.

Early diagnosis of acute adnexal torsion is vital in order to offer the possibility of conservative treatment. Delay in diagnosis exposes the patient to the risk of adnexal necrosis. However, in our series, the only feature significantly associated with adnexal necrosis was the presence of a large cyst measuring 150 mm [80-220].

In the light of these results, we emphasise the vital importance of early diagnosis of adnexal torsion, and believe that the rate of radical treatment could be reduced, to be limited only to masses suspected of malignancy or in menopausal women. Crelioscopy is currently the mainstay of diagnosis and treatment, which should be conservative as far as possible in order to preserve fertility.

6 BIBLIOGRAPHICAL REFERENCES

1. Melcer Y, Maymon R, Pekar-Zlotin M, Vaknin Z, Pansky M, Smorgick N. Does she have adnexal torsion? Prediction of adnexal torsion in reproductive age women. Arch Gynecol Obstet. March 2018;297(3):685-90.

2. Strachowski LM, Choi HH, Shum DJ, Horrow MM. Pearls and Pitfalls in Imaging of Pelvic Adnexal Torsion: Seven Tips to Tell It's Twisted. RadioGraphics. March 2021;41(2):625-40.

3. Ngo AV, Otjen JP, Parisi MT, Ferguson MR, Otto RK, Stanescu AL. Pediatric ovarian torsion: a pictorial review. Pediatr Radiol. Nov 2015;45(12):1845-55.

4. Sasaki KJ, Miller CE. Adnexal Torsion: Review of the Literature. Journal of Minimally Invasive Gynecology. March 2014;21(2):196-202.

5. Qian L. Isolated fallopian tube torsion with paraovarian cysts: a case report and literature review. 2021;7.

6. Melcer Y, Sarig-Meth T, Maymon R, Pansky M, Vaknin Z, Smorgick N. Similar But Different: A Comparison of Adnexal Torsion in Pediatric, Adolescent, and Pregnant and Reproductive-Age Women. Journal of Women's Health. Apr 2016;25(4):391-6.

7. Cohen A, Solomon N, Almog B, Cohen Y, Tsafrir Z, Rimon E, et al. Adnexal Torsion in Postmenopausal Women: Clinical Presentation and Risk of Ovarian Malignancy. Journal of Minimally Invasive Gynecology. jan 2017;24(1):94-7.

8. Chu K, Zhang Q, Sun N, Ding H, Li W. Conservative laparoscopic management of adnexal torsion based on a 17-year follow-up experience. J Int Med Res. Apr 2018;46(4):1685-9.

9. Glanc P, Ghandehari H, Kahn D, Melamed N. OP15.09: Acute ovarian torsion: the impact of time delays to surgery: OP15.09: Acute ovarian torsion: the impact of time delays to surgery. Ultrasound Obstet Gynecol. Sep 2015;46:99-99.

10. Ghulmiyyah L, Nassar A, Sassine D, Khoury S, Nassif J, Ramadan H, et al. Accuracy of Pelvic Ultrasound in Diagnosing Adnexal Torsion. Radiol Res Pract. 1 Jul 2019;2019:1406291.

11. Bardin R, Perl N, Mashiach R, Ram E, Orbach-Zinger S, Shmueli A, et al. Prediction of Adnexal Torsion by Ultrasound in Women with Acute Abdominal Pain. Ultraschall Med. Dec 2020;41(06):688-94.

12. Chang HC, Bhatt S, Dogra VS. Pearls and Pitfalls in Diagnosis of Ovarian Torsion. RadioGraphics. Sept 2008;28(5):1355-68.

13. Bronstein M, Pandya S, Snyder C, Shi Q, Muensterer O. A Meta-Analysis of B-Mode Ultrasound, Doppler Ultrasound, and Computed Tomography to

Diagnose Pediatric Ovarian Torsion. Eur J Pediatr Surg. 30 Aug 2014;25(01):82-6.
14. Mashiach R, Melamed N, Gilad N, Ben-Shitrit G, Meizner I. Sonographic Diagnosis of Ovarian Torsion: Accuracy and Predictive Factors. Journal of Ultrasound in Medicine. Sept 2011;30(9):1205-10.
15. Ssi-Yan-Kai G, Rivain AL, Trichot C, Morcelet MC, Prevot S, Deffieux X, et al. What every radiologist should know about adnexal torsion. Emerg Radiol. Feb 2018;25(1):51-9.
16. Grunau GL, Harris A, Buckley J, Todd NJ. Diagnosis of Ovarian Torsion: Is It Time to Forget About Doppler? Journal of Obstetrics and Gynaecology Canada. Jul 2018;40(7):871-5.
17. Robertson JJ, Long B, Koyfman A. Myths in the Evaluation and Management of Ovarian Torsion. The Journal of Emergency Medicine. Apr 2017;52(4):449-56.
18. Huchon C, Panel P, Kayem G, Schmitz T, Nguyen T, Fauconnier A. Does this woman have adnexal torsion? Human Reproduction. 1 Aug 2012;27(8):2359-64.
19. Chiesa-Vottero A. Risk of Malignancy in Postmenopausal Patients With Ovarian Torsion. International Journal of Gynecological Pathology. Jan 2020;39(1):e4.
20. Ganer Herman H, Shalev A, Ginat S, Kerner R, Keidar R, Bar J, et al. Clinical characteristics of adnexal torsion in premenarchal patients. Arch Gynecol Obstet. March 2016;293(3):603-8.
21. Rey-Bellet Gasser C, Gehri M, Joseph JM, Pauchard JY. Is It Ovarian Torsion? A Systematic Literature Review and Evaluation of Prediction Signs: Pediatric Emergency Care. Apr 2016;32(4):256-61.
22. Asfour V, Varma R, Menon P. Clinical risk factors for ovarian torsion. :6.
23. Ahui E A, Ke N, An K, A S, Jjk E, N K, et al. Echographic Etiological Diagnosis of Acute Pelvic Pain in Women in the Ivory Coast. ESJ [Internet]. 31 Jul 2019 [cite 14 Jul 2022]; 15(21). Available from: http://eujournal.org/index.php/esj/article/view/12262/11827
24. Yuk JS, Yang SW, Lee MH, Kyung MS. Incidence of Adnexal Torsion in the Republic of Korea: A Nationwide Serial Cross-Sectional Study (2009-2018). J Pers Med. 29 Jul 2021;11(8):743.
25. Huang C, Hong MK, Ding DC. A review of ovary torsion. Tzu Chi Med J. 2017;29(3):143.
26. Spinelli C, Piscioneri J, Strambi S. Adnexal torsion in adolescents: update

and review of the literature. Current Opinion in Obstetrics & Gynecology. oct 2015;27(5):320-5.
27. Alrabeeah A, Galliani CA, Giacomantonio M, Heifetz SA, Lau H. Neonatal Ovarian Torsion: Report of Three Cases and Review of the Literature. :7.
28. Otjen JP, Stanescu AL, Alessio AM, Parisi MT. Ovarian torsion: developing a machine-learned algorithm for diagnosis. Pediatr Radiol. May 2020;50(5):706-14.
29. Ogawa C, Amano T, Higuchi A, Tsuji S, Kimura F, Murakami T. Adnexal torsion without neoplastic lesions after laparoscopic hysterectomy: A report of three cases and literature review. J Obstet Gynaecol Res. Feb 2021;47(2):851-4.
30. Ashwal E, Hiersch L, Krissi H, Eitan R, Less S, Wiznitzer A, et al. Characteristics and Management of Ovarian Torsion in Premenarchal Compared With Postmenarchal Patients. Obstetrics & Gynecology. Sep 2015;126(3):514-20.
31. Feng JL, Lei T, Xie HN, Li LJ, Du L. Spectrums and Outcomes of Adnexal Torsion at Different Ages: Spectrums and Outcomes of Adnexal Torsion. J Ultrasound Med. Sep 2017;36(9):1859-66.
32. Resapu P, Rao Gundabattula S, Bharathi Bayyarapu V, Pochiraju M, Surampudi K, Dasari S. Adnexal torsion in symptomatic women: a single-centre retrospective study of diagnosis and management. Journal of Obstetrics and Gynaecology. Apr 3, 2019;39(3):349-54.
33. Moro F, Bolomini G, Sibal M, Vijayaraghavan SB, Venkatesh P, Nardelli F, et al. Imaging in gynecological disease (20): clinical and ultrasound characteristics of adnexal torsion. Ultrasound Obstet Gynecol. Dec 2020;56(6):934-43.
34. Duan N, Chen X, Rao M, Zhou C, Wang Z. CT predictive model for torsion angle as a marker for risk of necrosis in patients with adnexal torsion. Clinical Radiology. Jul 2021;76(7):540-6.
35. Guven S, Kart C, Guvendag Guven ES, Cetin EC, Mente§e A. Is the Measurement of Serum Ischemia-Modified Albumin the Best Test to Diagnose Ovarian Torsion? Gynecol Obstet Invest. 2015;79(4):269-75.
36. Gu X, Yang M, Liu Y, Liu F, Liu D, Shi F. The ultrasonic whirlpool sign combined with plasma d-dimer level in adnexal torsion. European Journal of Radiology. dec 2018;109:196-202.
37. Lee CH, Raman S, Sivanesaratnam V. Torsion of ovarian tumors: A clinicopathological study. International Journal of Gynecology & Obstetrics. Jan 1989;28(1):21-5.
38. Vijayalakshmi K, Reddy GMM, Subbiah VN, Sathiya S, Arjun B. Clinico-

Pathological Profile of Adnexal Torsion Cases: A Retrospective Analysis from A Tertiary Care Teaching Hospital. J Clin Diagn Res. June 2014;8(6):OC04-7.
39. Meyer R, Meller N, Komem DA, Tsur A, Cohen SB, Mashiach R, et al. Pregnancy outcomes following laparoscopy for suspected adnexal torsion during pregnancy. The Journal of Maternal-Fetal & Neonatal Medicine. 6 Jul 2021;1-7.
40. Nair S. Five Year Retrospective Case Series of Adnexal Torsion. JCDR [Internet]. 2014 [cite 26 Jul 2022]; Available from: http://jcdr.net/article_fulltext.asp?issn=0973-709x&year=2014&volume=8&issue=12&page=OC09&issn=0973-709x&id=5251
41. Meyer R, Meller N, Mohr-Sasson A, Toussia-Cohen S, Komem DA, Mashiach R, et al. A clinical prediction model for adnexal torsion in pediatric and adolescent population. Journal of Pediatric Surgery. March 2022;57(3):497-501.
42. Warwar RE, Schmidt GE. Bilateral ovarian torsion with ovarian fusion in the setting of polycystic ovarian syndrome: A case report. Case Reports in Women's Health. Jul 2019;23:e00129.
43. Dawood MT, Naik M, Bharwani N, Sudderuddin SA, Rockall AG, Stewart VR. Adnexal Torsion: Review of Radiologic Appearances. RadioGraphics. March 2021;41(2):609-24.
44. Huchon C, Staraci S, Fauconnier A. Adnexal torsion: a predictive score for pre-operative diagnosis. Human Reproduction. 1 Sep 2010;25(9):2276-80.
45. Hartley J, Akhtar M, Edi-Osagie E. Oophoropexy for Recurrent Ovarian Torsion. Case Rep Obstet Gynecol. 6 Feb 2018;2018:8784958.
46. Brady PC, Styer AK. Laparoscopic uteroovarian ligament truncation and uterosacral oophoropexy for idiopathic recurrent ovarian torsion: case report and review of literature. Fertil Res and Pract. dec 2015;1(1):2.
47. Dasgupta R, Renaud E, Goldin AB, Baird R, Cameron DB, Arnold MA, et al. Ovarian torsion in pediatric and adolescent patients: A systematic review. Journal of Pediatric Surgery. Jul 2018;53(7):1387-91.
48. Pansky M, Smorgick N, Herman A, Schneider D, Halperin R. Torsion of normal adnexa in postmenarchal women and risk of recurrence. Obstet Gynecol. Feb 2007;109(2 Pt 1):355-9.
49. Bitri M. Adnexal torsion a propos de 23 cases [These Med]. [Tunis]: Tunis; 1991.
50. Bar-On S, Mashiach R, Stockheim D, Soriano D, Goldenberg M, Schiff E, et al. Emergency laparoscopy for suspected ovarian torsion: are we too hasty to operate? Fertility and Sterility. Apr 2010;93(6):2012-5.

51. Adeyemi-Fowode O, McCracken KA, Todd NJ. Adnexal torsion. Journal of Pediatric and Adolescent Gynecology. august 2018;31(4):333 -8.
52. Wang Z, Zhang D, Zhang H, Guo X, Zheng J, Xie H. Characteristics of the patients with adnexal torsion and outcomes of different surgical procedures. Medicine (Baltimore). Feb 1, 2019;98(5):e14321.
53. Spinelli C, Piscioneri J, Strambi S. Adnexal torsion in adolescents: update and review of the literature. Current Opinion in Obstetrics & Gynecology. oct 2015;27(5):320-5.
54. Tzur T, Smorgick N, Sharon N, Pekar-Zlotin M, Maymon R, Melcer Y. Adnexal torsion with paraovarian cysts in pediatric and adolescent populations: A retrospective study. Journal of Pediatric Surgery. Feb 2021;56(2):324-7.
55. Korkmaz U, Bakir MS, Sagni? S, Simsek T. Chronic ovarian torsion after vaginal hysterectomy: a case with metastatic serous ovarian cancer. :7.
56. Bouguizane S, Bibi H, Farhat Y, Dhifallah S, Darraji F, Hidar S, et al [Adnexal torsion: a report of 135 cases]. J Gynecol Obstet Biol Reprod (Paris). Oct 2003;32(6):535-40.
57. Mazouni C, Bretelle F, Menard JP, Blanc B, Gamerre M. Diagnosis of adnexal torsion: are there predictive signs of necrosis? Gynecologie Obstetrique & Fertilite. March 2005;33(3):102-6.
58. Benkirane S, Alaoui FF, Chaara H, Bougern H, Melhouf MA. Twisted paratubal cyst: a rare case of difficult diagnosis. :4.
59. Bakacak M, Kostu B, Ercan O, Bostanci MS, Kiran G, Aral M, et al. High-sensitivity C-reactive protein as a novel marker in early diagnosis of ovarian torsion: an experimental study. Arch Gynecol Obstet. Jan 2015;291(1):99-104.
60. Wattar B, Rimmer M, Rogozinska E, Macmillian M, Khan K, Al Wattar B. Accuracy of imaging modalities for adnexal torsion: a systematic review and meta-analysis. BJOG: Int J Obstet Gy. Jan 2021;128(1):37 -44.
61. Ssi-Yan-Kai G, Rivain AL, Trichot C, Morcelet MC, Prevot S, Deffieux X, et al. What every radiologist should know about adnexal torsion. Emerg Radiol. Feb 2018;25(1):51-9.
62. Patil AR, Nandikoor S, Rao A, M Janardan G, Kheda A, Hari M, et al. Multimodality imaging in adnexal torsion: Adnexal torsion. Journal of Medical Imaging and Radiation Oncology. feb 2015;59(1):7-19.
63. Sibal M. Follicular Ring Sign: A Simple Sonographic Sign for Early Diagnosis of Ovarian Torsion. Journal of Ultrasound in Medicine. nov 2012;31(11):1803-9.
64. Bar-On S, Mashiach R, Stockheim D, Soriano D, Goldenberg M, Schiff E, et al. Emergency laparoscopy for suspected ovarian torsion: are we too hasty to

operate? Fertility and Sterility. Apr 2010;93(6):2012-5.
65. Valsky DV, Esh-Broder E, Cohen SM, Lipschuetz M, Yagel S. Added value of the gray-scale whirlpool sign in the diagnosis of adnexal torsion. Ultrasound in Obstetrics & Gynecology. 2010;36(5):630-4.
66. Raman Patil A, Nandikoor S, Chaitanya Reddy S. CT in the diagnosis of adnexal torsion: a retrospective study. Journal of Obstetrics and Gynaecology. 2 Apr 2020;40(3):388-94.
67. Mandoul C, Verheyden C, Curros-Doyon F, Rathat G, Taourel P, Millet I. Diagnostic performance of CT signs for predicting adnexal torsion in women presenting with an adnexal mass and abdominal pain: A case-control study. European Journal of Radiology. Jan 2018;98:75-81.
68. Lee MS, Moon MH, Woo H, Sung CK, Oh S, Jeon HW, et al. CT findings of adnexal torsion: A matched case-control study. Lagana AS, editor. PLoS ONE. 11 Jul 2018;13(7):e0200190.
69. Ling-Shan C, Jing L, Zheng-Qiu Z, Pin W, Zhi-Tao W, Fu-Ting T, et al. Computed Tomography Features of Adnexal Torsion: A Meta-Analysis. Academic Radiology. Feb 2022;29(2):317-25.
70. Duigenan S, Oliva E, Lee SI. Ovarian Torsion: Diagnostic Features on CT and MRI With Pathologic Correlation. American Journal of Roentgenology. Feb 2012;198(2):W122-31.
71. Swenson DW, Lourenco AP, Beaudoin FL, Grand DJ, Killelea AG, McGregor AJ. Ovarian torsion: Case-control study comparing the sensitivity and specificity of ultrasonography and computed tomography for diagnosis in the emergency department. European Journal of Radiology. Apr 2014;83(4):733-8.
72. Takeda A, Hayashi S, Teranishi Y, Imoto S, Nakamura H. Chronic adnexal torsion: An under-recognized disease entity. European Journal of Obstetrics & Gynecology and Reproductive Biology. march 2017;210:45-53.
73. Fei Y, Quint E, Rosen M, Dendrinos M. 48. Chronic Adnexal Torsion Presenting as Intermittent Pelvic Pain. Journal of Pediatric and Adolescent Gynecology. Apr 2021;34(2):258.
74. Ito F. Isolated fallopian tube torsion diagnosed and treated with laparoscopic surgery: A case report. Gynecology and Minimally Invasive Therapy. 2017;3.
75. Hagege R. Isolated Fallopian Tube Torsion: An Underdiagnosed Entity with Debatable Management. 2021;00(00):6.
76. Gulino FA, Ettore C, Morreale G, Siringo S, Russo E, D'Asta M, et al. Isolated Tubal Torsion in a Term Pregnancy: Case Report and Systematic Review of

Literature of the Last 10 Years. Front Surg. 5 Apr 2022;9:856915.
77. Blitz MJ, Appelbaum H. Torsion of Fallopian Tube Remnant Associated with Noncommunicating Rudimentary Horn in Adolescent Girl with Unicornuate Uterus. Journal of Pediatric and Adolescent Gynecology. oct 2014;27(5):e97-9.
78. Shevach Alon A, Kerner R, Ginath S, Barda G, Bar J, Sagiv R. Clinical Characteristics of Women with Isolated Fallopian Tube Torsion Compared with Adnexal Torsion. Isr Med Assoc J. Sep 2019;21(9):575-9.
79. Bharathi A, Gowri M. Torsion of the Fallopian Tube and the Haematosalpinx in Perimenopausal Women- A Case Report. J Clin Diagn Res. Apr 2013;7(4):731-3.
80. Kartal T, Birge O. Bilateral torsion of fallopian tubes with bilateral hydrosalpinx: a case report. J Med Case Rep. 5 August 2020;14:120.
81. Adnexal torsion on paratubal cyst: report of a rare case - ProQuest [Internet]. Available on [cite 25 aout2022] : https://www.proquest.com/openview/9d2cdd98ee80dd7e84cccd88b7b68f66/1?pq-origsite=gscholar&cbl=2031961
82. Baradwan S, Sendy W, Sendy S. Bilateral dermoid ovarian torsion in a young woman: a case report. J Med Case Reports. Dec 2018;12(1):159.
83. Kurtoglu E, Kokcu A, Danaci M. Asynchronous Bilateral Ovarian Torsion. A Case Report and Mini Review. Journal of Pediatric and Adolescent Gynecology. june 2014;27(3):122-4.
84. Lucchetti MC, Orazi C, Lais A, Capitanucci ML, Caione P, Bakhsh H. Asynchronous Bilateral Ovarian Torsion: Three Cases, Three Lessons. Case Rep Pediatr. 2017;2017:6145467.
85. Raicevic M, Saxena AK. Asynchronus bilateral ovarian torsions in girls-systematic review. World J Pediatr. oct 2017;13(5):416-20.
86. Department of Obstetrics and Gynecology, Bursa Yuksek Ihtisas Training and Research Hospital, Bursa, Turkey, Dincgez Cakmak B, Ozgen G, Department of Obstetrics and Gynecology, Bursa Yuksek Ihtisas Training and Research Hospital, Bursa, Turkey, Dundar B, Department of Obstetrics and Gynecology, Bursa Yuksek Ihtisas Training and Research Hospital, Bursa, Turkey, et al. Management of Bilateral Adnexal Torsion in a Case of Ovarian Hyperstimulation Syndrome. Eur Arch Med Res. 14 Sep 2018;34(3):196-9.
87. Souabni SA, Belhaddad EH. Large bilateral ovarian cysts with left ovarian torsion and right dermoid cyst. Pan Afr Med J. 29 Oct 2020;37:191.
88. Guennoun A, Krimou Y, Mamouni N, Errarhay S, Bouchikhi C, Banani A. Healthy adnexal torsion and pregnancy: a case report. Pan Afr Med J [Internet].

2017 [cited 28 Aug 2022];27. Available from: http://www.panafrican-med-journal.com/content/article/27/197/full/

89. Ayachi A, Blel Z, Khelifa N, Mkaouer L, Bouchahda R, Mourali M. Adnexal torsion in the second trimester of pregnancy, a propos de deux cas. Pan Afr Med J [Internet]. 2016 [cited 14 Jul 2022];25. Available from: http://www.panafrican- med-journal.com/content/article/25/113/full/

90. Karrer FW. Twisted Ovarian Cyst in a Newborn Infant: Report of a Case. Arch Surg. 1 Dec 1961;83(6):921.

91. M M, F S, B S, KM. Ovarian torsion causing bowel obstruction in a premature infant. Journal of Pediatric Surgery Case Reports. 1 Sep 2022;84:102381.

92. Joshi J, Kamath N, Kini JR, K J, Rao S, Kamath SP. Antenatal Ovarian Torsion Presenting With Features of Intestinal Obstruction in a Neonate. Journal of Nepal Paediatric Society. 15 Dec 2020;40(3):265-9.

93. Toker Kurtmen B, Divarci E, Ergun O, Ozok G, Celik A. The Role of Surgery in Antenatal Ovarian Torsion: Retrospective Evaluation of 28 Cases and Review of the Literature. Journal of Pediatric and Adolescent Gynecology. 1 Feb 2022;35(1):18-22.

94. Saeed H, Hong L, Smith N, Shaman M. Ovarian torsion in utero diagnosed at 37 weeks of pregnancy: A case report. Case Reports in Women's Health. 1 Jul 2020;27:e00232.

95. Hasson J, Tsafrir Z, Azem F, Bar-On S, Almog B, Mashiach R, et al. Comparison of adnexal torsion between pregnant and nonpregnant women. American Journal of Obstetrics and Gynecology. June 2010;202(6):536.e1-536.e6.

96. Hua D, Zhao P, Jiang L. Torsion of ovarian endometrioma in pregnancy: a case report and review of the literature. Trop Doct. Jul 2019;49(3):221-3.

97. Yu M, Liu Y, Jia D, Tian T, Xi Q. Adnexal torsion in pregnancy after in vitro fertilization. Medicine (Baltimore). 22 Jan 2021;100(3):e24009.

98. Fouedjio JH, Fouogue JT, Fouelifack FY, Nangue C, Sando Z, Mbu RE. Adnexal torsion during pregnancy: a case report from Yaounde Central Hospital, Cameroon. Pan Afr Med J [Internet]. 2014 [cited 5 June 2022];17. Available at: http://www.panafrican-med-journal.com/content/article/17/39/full/

99. Wang Y xue, Deng S. Clinical characteristics, treatment and outcomes of adnexal torsion in pregnant women: a retrospective study. BMC Pregnancy Childbirth. Dec 2020;20(1):483.

100. Dvash S, Pekar M, Melcer Y, Weiner Y, Vaknin Z, Smorgick N. Adnexal Torsion in Pregnancy Managed by Laparoscopy Is Associated with Favorable Obstetric Outcomes. Journal of Minimally Invasive Gynecology. Sept 2020;27(6):1295-9.
101. Kahramanoglu I, Eroglu V, Turan H, Kaval G, Sal V, Tokgozoglu N. Isolated adnexal torsion in a 20-week spontaneous twin pregnancy. International Journal of Surgery Case Reports. 2016;23:138-40.
102. Bernigaud O, Fraison E, Thiberville G, Lamblin G. Ovarian torsion in a twin pregnancy at 32 weeks and 6 days: A case-report. Journal of Gynecology Obstetrics and Human Reproduction. June 2021;50(6):102117.
103. Chateil JF, Eresue-Bony M, Gautier R. Evaluer la dose efficace delivree en radiographie conventionnelle et en tomodensitometrie. Journal of diagnostic and interventional imaging. Sep 1, 2019;2(4):176-81.
104. Cunha S, Coutada R, Neiva AR, Goncalves E, Pinheiro P. Adnexal torsion in post-menopausal women: an even more challenging diagnosis. Prog obstet ginecol (Ed impr). 2018;48-51.
105. Parker WH. Bilateral oophorectomy versus ovarian conservation: effects on long-term women's health. J Minim Invasive Gynecol. Apr 2010;17(2):161 -6.
106. Kives S, Gascon S, Dubuc E, Van Eyk N. No. 341-Diagnosis and Management of Adnexal Torsion in Children, Adolescents, and Adults. Journal of Obstetrics and Gynaecology Canada. feb 2017;39(2):82-90.
107. Michelis LD, Politch JA, Kuohung W. Factors Associated with Oophorectomy in Patients with Suspected Ovarian Torsion. Journal of Gynecologic Surgery. 1 June 2021;37(3):236-40.
108. Zangene M, Ashoori Barmchi A, Rezaei M, Veisi F. The comparison between the serum level of interleukin-6 in women with acute ovarian torsion and other causes of lower abdominal pain. Journal of Obstetrics and Gynaecology. 18 Oct 2016;1-5.
109. Ganesh D, Rajkumar A, Rajkumar JS, Guru V. Ruptured Ectopic Pregnancy with Contralateral Ovarian Serous Cyst Adenoma Torsion: Laparoscopic Management of Double Trouble. Case Reports in Obstetrics and Gynecology. 2016;2016:1-3.
110. Kaya C, Ekin M, Cengiz H, Yasar L, dogan K. A Rare Case: Ruptured Ectopic Pregnancy with Contralateral Adnexal Torsion. Bakirkoy Tip Dergisi. March 27, 2015;11:29-32.
111. Sendy S, Abuy A, Sendy W, Baradwan S. Unusual presentation of bilateral pyosalpinx mimicking an ovarian torsion: A case report. Ann Med Surg (Lond).

26 Feb 2020;52:16-8.

112. Akata D. Ovarian Torsion and Its Mimics. Ultrasound Clinics. July 2008;3(3):451-60.

113. Le D, Dey CB, Byun K. Imaging findings of a torsed pedunculated uterine leiomyoma: A case report. Radiol Case Rep. 28 Nov 2019;15(2):144-9.

114. Timmons D, Montrief T, Koyfman A, Long B. Ovarian hyperstimulation syndrome: A review for emergency clinicians. The American Journal of Emergency Medicine. August 2019;37(8):1577-84.

7 APPENDICES

Appendix 1: Data collection form

Index : Personnel number :

File number : Year :

Phone number :

Consultation date : Consultation time :

Date of admission : Admission time :

Last name: First name :

Anamnese:

Age:

Medical history: Fx :

Mx :

Chx :

G/O : young girl : yes / No

G P A

History of cyst :

History of cystectomy :

History of adnexal torsion :

Pregnant: Yes / No

Scarred uterus: yes/no

DDR :

Reason for consultation :

Clinical picture :

General condition :

TA : FC :

Temperature :

Pain: Time of onset

Time between onset of pain and consultation:

Mode of installation :

Broadcast :

Similar previous episode:

Associated signs :

Digestive signs : Nausea :Vomiting :

Urinary signs :

Physical examination :

Location:

Presence of pelvic mass: yes / no

Speculum examination: neck: macroscopic appearance :

Leucorrhee :

If yes: Appearance

Abondance

Odour

Bleeding :

If yes: Spontaneous contact

IUD thread :

VT: pain on uterine mobilisation:

Douglas CDS pain: right left bilateral

Biology :

CRP :

GB :

Beta HCG :

Ultrasound: suprapubic : Endovaginal :

Uterus :

Ovary increases in size: yes / no

Hyperechogenic stroma: yes / no

Peripheral arrangement of follicles: yes / no

Cyst: Number :

Location:

Size :

Echogenicite :

Contents:

Partition :

Vegetation :

Doppler study: done / not done

If done :

Vascularisation of the adnexa: present / reduced / absent

Whirlpool sign : present / no

Douglas effusion: yes / no

Abondance :

Others :

CT scan done: yes / no

If done: signs of torsion :

Surgery :

Time of admission :

Time of transfer to operating theatre :

Route: Laparotomy / Laparoscopy / Conversion

Effusion: yes / No

Torsion pressure: yes / no

If Twisted: Number of turns :

Torsion dimension :

Torsion seat :

Twisted appendix :

Associated adnexal pathology: yes / no

If yes: Size

Content

Status of the controlateral appendix :

If no torsion: other diagnosis:

Action taken :

Intraoperative complications :

Intraoperative cytology: yes / no

Post-operative follow-up :

Complications :

Release date :

Progression of the pregnancy :

Anatomopathological findings :

TITLE

Adnexal torsion: experience of the Monastir maternity and neonatology centre

SUMMARY

Introduction: Adnexal torsion is a gynaecological emergency of multifactorial pathogenesis. The clinical expression is polymorphous and the imaging examinations are generally non-specific. The aim of our study is to determine the various **clinical and para-clinical** signs **of adnexal torsion, as well as the prognostic factors**, and to establish a clinical-biological, radiological and peroperative comparison of patients **presenting with adnexal torsion**.

Methods: This is a retrospective descriptive and analytical study carried out in the gynecology and obstetrics **department** of the Monastir maternity and neonatology centre over a 5-year **period** from 1 January 2017 to 31 January 2022.

Results: For 106 patients presenting with adnexal torsion, the diagnosis was confirmed surgically in 66 patients. **The mean age of our** patients was 25.92±9.09 years, with extremes ranging from 13 to 53 years. The **age** group most affected was 20 to 30 years. Thirty-seven patients were single and thirty-nine patients were nulliparous. 48.4% of patients consulted during the follicular phase, which was significantly associated with torsion. Sudden pelvic pain (71.7%), localised (75%) and on the right (42.4%), dominated the clinical picture. Vomiting, present in 41.7% of cases, was significantly associated with torsion. **Hyperleukocytosis (>10000 E/mm3) and elevated CRP (>5mg/L)** were **not significantly associated with torsion. Pelvic ultrasound was performed in all our patients. An enlarged ovary was noted in 56.7%** of cases. The presence of an adnexal mass was significantly associated with **adnexal** torsion. **Cysts larger than 5 cm, with anechogenic contents, dermoid appearance** or paratubal location were significantly associated with torsion, in contrast to cysts with hyperechogenic contents or a **hemorrhagic cyst appearance. The** differential diagnoses of the remaining 40 patients were dominated by **hemorrhagic** corpus **luteum** cysts **(13 cases) and uncomplicated benign ovarian cysts (9 cases).** Utero-annexal infections were **found in 4 cases and acute appendicitis in 2 cases. No diagnosis was found in 2 patients. Laparoscopy was used to diagnose torsion in 61.7% of cases, and conservative treatment of the twisted adnexa was** performed in 88.3% of cases.

Conclusion: In the light of our results, we emphasise the need for a systematic gynaecological **examination** coupled with pelvic ultrasound in any woman presenting with **acute pelvic pain, and that the presence of an adnexal mass** in this context will indicate **the need for emergency crelioscopy, which would enable a precise diagnosis and offer the possibility of conservative treatment in order to preserve the patient's fertility.**

KEYWORDS: |[

ouleur, Kyste, Annexes, Torsion, Ischemie, Fertilite

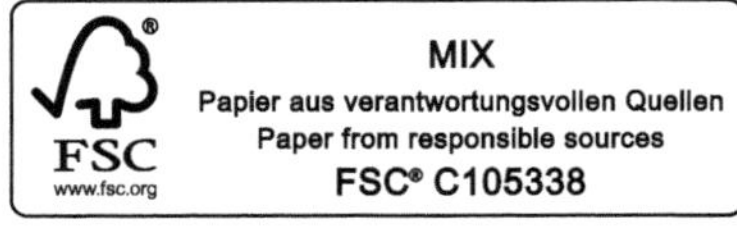

Printed by Books on Demand GmbH, Norderstedt / Germany